ANNUAL REVIEW OF NURSING RESEARCH

Volume 5, 1987

ANNUAL REVIEW OF NURSING RESEARCH

Volume 5, 1987

Joyce J. Fitzpatrick, Ph.D.
Roma Lee Taunton, Ph.D.
Editors

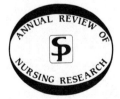

SPRINGER PUBLISHING COMPANY
New York

Order ANNUAL REVIEW OF NURSING RESEARCH, Volume 6, 1988, prior to publication and receive a 10% discount. An order coupon can be found after the index.

Springer Publishing Company, Inc.
536 Broadway
New York, NY 10012

87 88 89 90 91 / 5 4 3 2 1

ISBN 0-8261-4354-7
ISSN 0739-6686

ANNUAL REVIEW OF NURSING RESEARCH is indexed in *Cumulative Index to Nursing and Allied Health Literature* and *Index Medicus*.

Printed in the United States of America

Contents

Publisher's Note

This volume marks an important transition in the life of the *Annual Review of Nursing Research*. Dr. Harriet Werley, who with characteristic energy and inspiration founded the Review, has with this volume stepped down from its editorship. She will remain actively involved as a member of the Advisory Board. We wish to express our grateful appreciation to her for the groundbreaking and very successful work that she has done in planning and editing the Review over the years.

The editorial leadership remains in the capable hands of Dr. Joyce Fitzpatrick, who has skillfully co-edited the Review from its inception, and Dr. Roma Lee Taunton, who came on board as a co-editor for Volume 4. Both distinguished scholars, they share Dr. Werley's vision of a rigorous forum for the best in nursing scholarship. This volume represents a proud continuation of that vision.

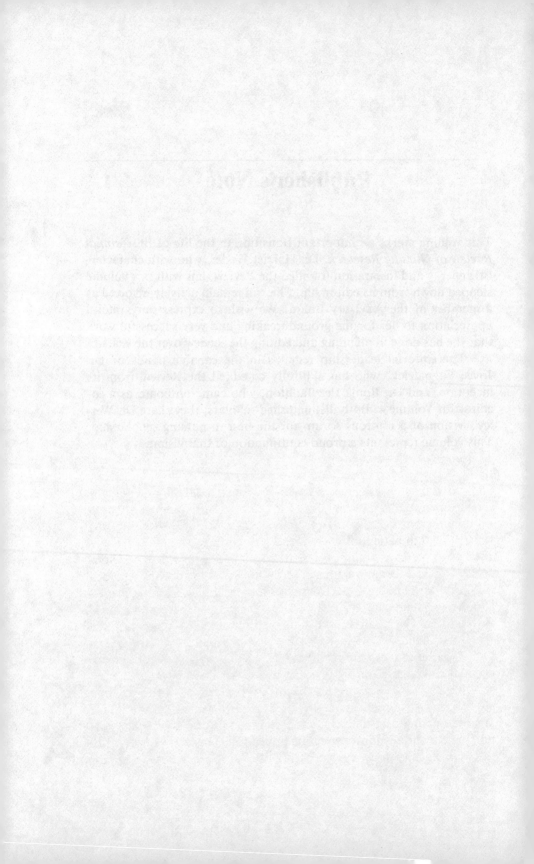

Preface

This is the fifth volume in the *Annual Review of Nursing Research (ARNR)* series. Volume 1 appeared in December 1983; Volume 2 in October 1984; Volume 3 in May 1985; and Volume 4 in April 1986; this volume will appear in early 1987. Volumes 6 through 8 currently are in the planning and production stages, and soon we will be initiating discussions with potential authors for future volumes.

We have received a very positive response from the scientific community regarding the launching of this landmark series. We have introduced our work at various forums through presentations, symposia, and posters. Many of our colleagues have indicated that the *ARNR* series is a significant addition to their libraries. Importantly, we have received much positive feedback regarding the contribution of this series to the development of nursing knowledge for the discipline.

The chapters under Nursing Practice for Volume 5 pertain to human responses to actual and potential health problems. Volumes 1 and 4 chapters in this area were focused on human development along the life span, Volume 2 chapters on the family, and Volume 3 chapters on the community. Volume 6 chapters will address nursing interventions related to patient or client responses to health.

As in previous volumes, research reviewed for Volume 5 follows the established format of four other major parts in addition to Nursing Practice: Nursing Care Delivery, Nursing Education, the Profession of Nursing, and Other Research. In the nursing practice area, with a focus on human responses to health problems, Brenda L. Lyon and Joan Stehle Werner review ten years of research on stress, Ann Gill Taylor examines pain research, and Geraldene Felton reviews two decades of research on biologic rhythms. Mi Ja Kim introduces research on physiological responses in health and illness, which will be a specific thrust for the Nursing Practice area in Volumes 7 and 8. In the area of nursing care delivery, Kathleen Dracup presents critical care nursing. In the section on nursing education, Grace H. Chickadonz discusses faculty practice, and Christine A. Tanner deals with the teaching of clinical judgment. Research on the profession of nursing includes a chapter by Joanne Comi McCloskey and Marilyn T. Molen, who examine leadership in nursing. In the area of other research, Afaf Ibrahim Meleis's report on international nursing research is a continuation of our effort to include a chapter on nursing research in other countries, in this case across countries. Mary Cipriano Silva also contributed a chapter in the area of other research, presenting research based on conceptual models of nursing.

We acknowledge most gratefully the work of the authors, the advice and involvement of the Advisory Board members, the critiques of anonymous reviewers, and the editorial and clerical assistance provided by Lois Schweitzer at Case Western Reserve University and Lavonne Meyers at the University of Kansas. Further, we are indebted particularly to Nikki S. Polis, Ph.D. candidate at Case Western Reserve University, for her continued editorial assistance throughout the production of this volume.

We welcome readers' comments and suggestions for shaping the upcoming volumes, including identifying potential chapter contributors. Authors should be recognized authorities in their areas, who have completed significant research. Please let us know your interests.

Contributors

Grace H. Chickadonz, Ph.D.
School of Nursing
Medical College of Ohio
Toledo, Ohio

Kathleen Dracup, D.N.S.
School of Nursing
University of California-Los Angeles
Los Angeles, California

Geraldene Felton, Ph.D.
College of Nursing
University of Iowa
Iowa City, Iowa

Mi Ja Kim, Ph.D.
College of Nursing
University of Illinois at Chicago
Chicago, Illinois

Brenda L. Lyon, D.N.Sc.
School of Nursing
Indiana University
Indianapolis, Indiana

Joanne Comi McCloskey, Ph.D.
College of Nursing
University of Iowa
Iowa City, Iowa

Afaf Ibrahim Meleis, Ph.D.
School of Nursing
University of California-San Francisco
San Francisco, California

Marilyn T. Molen, Ph.D.
Bachelor of Arts in Nursing Program
Metropolitan State University
St. Paul, Minnesota

Mary Cipriano Silva, Ph.D.
School of Nursing
George Mason University
Fairfax, Virginia

Christine A. Tanner, Ph.D.
School of Nursing
Oregon Health Sciences University
Portland, Oregon

Ann Gill Taylor, Ed.D.
School of Nursing
University of Virginia
Charlottesville, Virginia

Joan Stehle Werner, Ph.D.
School of Nursing
University of Wisconsin-Eau Claire
Eau Claire, Wisconsin

Forthcoming

ANNUAL REVIEW OF
NURSING RESEARCH, Volume 6

Tentative Contents

PART I
Research on Nursing Practice

Chapter 1

Stress

BRENDA L. LYON
SCHOOL OF NURSING
INDIANA UNIVERSITY
AND
JOAN STEHLE WERNER
SCHOOL OF NURSING
UNIVERSITY OF WISCONSIN—EAU CLAIRE

CONTENTS

Stress is recognized widely by nurses as a practice-relevant phenomenon, yet it is a concept about which there is little theoretical and practical agreement. It is readily apparent from the 976 stress-related articles appearing in nursing journals since 1956 that the term "stress" is used with various definitions to represent a wide range of problems

The authors wish to recognize Cathy Faulstich, Sheila Scott, Rosalee Dyke, Jo Straneva, Mary McGuire, Barbara Mehring, Julie Radovan, and Clara Ronnerud for their invaluable assistance with the literature search and preliminary analysis.

and situations. Although the first indexed reference to stress appeared in the *Cumulative Index to Nursing and Allied Health Literature* (CINAHL) in 1956, nurses' interest in stress as a phenomenon for study has flourished since 1970.

This review was limited to research conducted by nurses and published from 1974 to 1984. Only studies of adults with the word "stress" in the title or with stress in the theoretical framework were reviewed. Computer searches and the CINAHL were used to identify studies. There were 82 studies identified that met the review criteria.

The critical review that follows was guided by the belief that the credibility of nursing science will, in large part, depend on the utility of the theoretical underpinnings and empirical generalizations that characterize nursing practice. Therefore, the purpose of the review was to evaluate both nurse researchers' conceptualizations of stress and their systematic inquiry into the phenomenon.

The vast majority of the studies reviewed had common and serious flaws that limited contributions to nursing science. To highlight the problems, the chapter was organized around theoretically distinct conceptualizations of stress and common measurement and methodological flaws. The critique is presented in a summary format citing representative studies as illustrative examples.

DEFINITIONS AND THEORETICAL ORIENTATIONS

The 82 studies were categorized into the following four theoretical orientations: (a) stress as a stimulus; (b) stress as a response; (c) stress as a transaction; and (d) atheoretical. The studies were fairly evenly distributed among the categories as follows: (a) 23 studies or 28% used a stimulus definition; (b) 20 studies or 24% used a response definition; (c) 17 studies or 21% used a transactional definition; and (d) 22 studies or 27% were atheoretical.

Stress as a Stimulus

When stress is defined as a stimulus it is conceptualized as causing a disrupted response. Historically the stimulus orientation had its roots in the works of Holmes and Masuda (1966) and Holmes and Rahe

(1967), which were focused on the development of the tool known as the Social Readjustment Rating Scale (SRRS) or Schedule of Recent Experiences (SRE). The tools were developed to measure the effects of significant life changes on health. In the early 1970s, Holmes and Rahe made an important semantic shift from the concept of change to the concept of stress, and consequently, they assumed that the SRRS or SRE measured stress in the form of life changes or life events.

The primary theoretical relationship proposed by the stimulus model is that too many life changes increase vulnerability to illness. Critical assumptions underlying the stimulus model of stress include (a) that life change events are normative and result in the same expenditure of "adaptation units" across time and across people; (b) that a person's perception of the event as positively toned or negatively toned is irrelevant; and (c) that there is a common threshold beyond which disruption occurs. The assumptions form the framework for a model that depicts the person as a passive recipient of stress. Stress is viewed as a stable, additive phenomenon that is measurable by researcher-selected life events that have preassigned normative weights derived from mean scores. The stress score is obtained by summing the weighted responses or by simply counting the events that have occurred (Rahe, 1977).

Stress was defined in the stimulus-based nursing studies as life change or life events. In quasi-experimental studies researchers hypothesized that life change influenced the perception of the severity of illness (Anderson & Pleticha, 1974); disruptions in blood pressure, heart rate, and stroke volume (Volicer & Volicer, 1977); seriousness of illness (Mishel, 1984); and the occurrence of electrocardiogram abnormalities (Haughey, Brasure, Maloney, & Graham, 1984). Studies have been conducted to develop tools modeled after the SRE for medical–surgical patients (Volicer, 1974, 1977; Volicer & Bohannon, 1975) and surgical intensive-care-unit patients (Ballard, 1981).

If stress is defined as a stimulus, important philosophical, theoretical, and measurement dilemmas must be addressed. The first dilemma, and perhaps the most fundamental philosophical one, is the lack of fit between a stimulus orientation and nursing's orientation to human experiences. Contrary to the assumptions inherent in the stimulus model, nursing as a discipline views human experiences as arising out of dynamic person–environment transactions and is focused on the individualized health-care needs of people. The philosophical dilemma here is that the assumptions inherent in the stimulus model are not compatible with nursing's assumptions about human experiences.

The second dilemma pertains to logical and empirical adequacy of the theoretical relationship proposed by advocates of the stimulus orientation. One of the criteria for logical adequacy is that accurate predictions can be made (Hardy, 1974; Walker & Avant, 1983). Nurse researchers who investigated the relationship between life events and some type of physical or mental disruption, had equivocal results; when relationships were found they were small in magnitude ($r = .20$ to .28). It is interesting to note that Jalowiec and Powers (1981) did not find a relationship between hypertensive and emergency room patients' ratings of their stress level and the number of life events experienced. Such findings are not surprising when the theoretical relationship postulated between life events and illness is based on the assumption that events affect people in the same way, irrespective of how the event is perceived by the person—an assumption that belies our current knowledge (Kobasa, 1979; Kobasa, Maddi, & Kan, 1982).

Perhaps the simplistic stimulus model is attractive to many nurse researchers because of their desire to find a composite tool that would be easy to administer. Use of such a tool to measure stress highlights the third dilemma, that of measurement. Measurement of stress as a stimulus in nursing research has involved the use of unidimensional tools such as the SRRS (Anderson & Pleticha, 1974; Beard, 1982), Schedule of Life Experiences (Jalowiec & Powers, 1981), and the Hospital Stress Rating Scale (HSRS) (Ballard, 1981; Volicer, 1977; Volicer & Bohannon, 1975; Volicer & Volicer, 1977). The dimensions typically used in nursing research have been either adaptation units, as used in the SRRS, or stressfulness, as used in the HSRS. Use of a unidimensional tool to measure stress oversimplifies a complex and not-well-defined construct. The unidimensional measurement negates other dimensions that may play an important role in whether or not a person experiences stress in an event context, such as negative or positive tone, controllability, predictability, and impact. An additional measurement problem is that typically the unidimensional event tool uses preestablished values based on the mean scores of previously studied populations to determine an index of stress. Reliance on group means as indicators of individual experiences obscures variability.

Volicer and Bohannon (1975) found a high degree of consensus among medical–surgical patients when they ranked hospital events on the dimension of stressfulness using a card sort procedure with low, medium, and high levels of stressfulness. It is not surprising that a high degree of agreement was obtained, given that individual differences in perceptions of a situation diminish when the situation is one that is commonly considered dangerous, for instance, hospitalization, fire, or disaster (Lazarus, 1966). However, even in these situations there will still remain some variations in perception or meaning of a situation. For example, it is quite possible that many, if not all, of the events identified in the HSRS would be perceived by some patients at some time as nonstressful. Although Volicer relied heavily on a model that we view as incompatible with nursing's focus, it is important to recognize that her work was the only program of stress research identified in the nursing literature.

Stress as a Response

When stress is defined as a response, it represents the disruption caused by a noxious stimulus or stressor. In the response model, therefore, stress is the dependent variable rather than the independent variable as in the stimulus model. The theory most commonly used by nurse researchers is the work of Selye (1956, 1976). Stress is defined in the response model as a nonspecific response of the body to demands placed on it (Selye, 1956, 1976). In other words, regardless of the cause, situational context, or psychological interpretation of a demanding situation, the stress response is characterized by the same chain of events and the same pattern of physiological correlates.

Stress in the response-based nursing studies was operationalized commonly by both physiological and psychological measures. Physiological measures included vital signs (Guzzeta & Forsyth, 1979), urinary Na/K ratio and 17-ketosteroids (Farr, Keene, Samson, & Michael, 1984), and cardiovascular complaints (Schwartz & Brenner, 1979). The most common psychological measurements included negatively toned emotions such as anxiety (Guzzetta & Forsyth, 1979).

Most researchers using the response model in quasi-experimental studies investigated the effects of an independent variable such as information (Toth, 1980), relaxation (Tamez, Moore, & Brown, 1978), or interpersonal interaction (Schwartz & Brenner, 1979) on the dependent variable of stress, inferred from both physiological and psychological indices. It was interesting to note that the independent variables in the response-based studies were most commonly nursing measures that were purported to mediate between the stressor, which was commonly assumed to be hospitalization, and the stress response. No theoretical explanations were offered regarding the cognitive mediating variables even though use of such variables is contrary to Selye's theory and empirical generalizations. Although Selye acknowledged the critical role of perception in psychological stress experiences in the late 1970s, he did not modify his theoretical explanations and maintained that stress was a nonspecific syndrome represented as the General Adaptation Syndrome.

Like the stimulus model of stress, the response model does not allow for individual differences in response patterns. The response model, therefore, like the stimulus model, is not considered to be compatible with nursing's view of human experiences.

Stress as a Transaction

When stress is defined as a transaction it is viewed as a concept that has heuristic value but in itself cannot be measured. Stress is a concept that encompasses a set of cognitive, affective, and adaptational (coping) variables that arise out of person–environment transactions. The person and environment are seen as constantly intertwined, each affecting the other and being affected by the other (Lazarus, 1966).

The assumptions central to the transactional approach include (a) stress is not measurable as a singular concept; and (b) cognitive appraisal mediates stress experiences. Unlike the stimulus and response models, the transactional model allows for individual differences and does not necessitate a normative approach to research.

When defined in the studies reviewed, stress was defined as a construct designating a broad class of experiences characterized by a demanding situation that taxes a person's resources or coping capabilities and evokes a negative affect (Bedsworth & Molen, 1982). As such, the word stress described a negatively toned experience that was inclusive of perceived demands and resources, cognitive appraisals, emotions, and coping responses. Often the definition of stress was not included in the research report or was not clear (Murphy, 1984). Unlike the research based on either the stimulus or response model, the transactional orientation necessitated that the researcher clearly delineate which aspects of the person–environment transaction were to be studied, for example, mood state or coping. It was perhaps for this reason that the researchers focused primarily on defining the independent and dependent variables and often did not include a definition of stress.

Most of the transaction studies were quasi-experimental in nature. The independent variables commonly represented a cognitive or instructional intervention to prepare a person for surgery (Foster, 1974; Hoffman, Donckers, & Hauser, 1978; Nolan, 1977; Sime, 1976).The dependent variables used in the studies cited included negatively toned affects such as anxiety, fear, anger, and depression, and recovery variables such as length of stay. Unlike the studies on coping reviewed by J. E. Johnson (1984), the studies reviewed here cited transaction-oriented stress theory as contributing to the theoretical framework of the study.

There were a few descriptive studies based on the transactional framework, such as the work of Bedsworth and Molen (1982). The purpose of the study was to describe psychological stress reported by spouses of myocardial infarction patients. The study provided a good example of consistency between theoretical framework and conceptual and operational definitions. Threat was defined conceptually as a state in which the individual anticipates a confrontation with a harmful condition of some sort. Further, it was operationalized as a verbal self-reported response to the question, "In dealing with this situation, what have you been most anxious . . . apprehensive . . . concerned . . . or worried about?" (p. 452).

Since 1980 there have been several researchers investigating life stress that represent a continuing interest in life events but in a transactional framework (Murphy, 1984; Norbeck, 1984; Tilden, 1983). As a transactional measure of stress-related variables, investigators typically have used the Life Experiences Survey (LES) (J. H. Johnson & Sarason, 1979; Sarason, Johnson, & Siegel, 1978), which permits the subject to evaluate both the tone of the event as positive or negative and the impact of the event.

The transactional orientation to stress is consistent with nursing's view of human experiences and permits the researcher to focus on individual differences in stress experiences. There are insufficient replications of studies to evaluate the cumulative results of research using the transactional orientation. However, it is possible to say that the approach does lend itself well to the identification of mediating variables that might be amenable to nursing intervention.

Atheoretical

A large number of the studies reviewed (22) were atheoretical, that is, were without a theoretical framework and definition of stress (i.e., Hoffman et al., 1978; Miller & Grim, 1979) or had incompatible theoretical and operational definitions (Bell, 1977; Foster, 1974). Incompatible definitions suggested a lack of a sound theoretical foundation. The study conducted by Scott, Oberst, and Bookbinder (1984) was an example of incompatibility because stress was defined in the transactional framework (an individualized, cognitively mediated experience) but was measured using the normative, stimulus-based SRRS.

The studies were divided evenly between descriptive and quasi-experimental. The descriptive studies typically elicited types of situations or events that patients found to be stressful (i.e., Volicer, 1974). Investigators used dependent variables in quasi-experimental studies that were similar to those used in studies based on a transactional framework, including anxiety (Guzzeta, 1979); depression, anger, and fear (Schwartz & Brenner, 1979); coping (Bell, 1977); and vocal muscle tension (Fuller & Foster, 1982). Guzzeta also used a similar independent variable, information. The greatest weakness of the atheoretical studies was that there could be no direct contribution to nursing science through theory testing.

VALIDITY ISSUES

A major area of concern with the studies reviewed was that of validity. None of the stress studies were strictly basic, that is, contribution to law-like principles was not the objective. Roughly 40% of the studies were quasi-experimental, ex post facto, or causal comparative in nature. Because the construct of causality was the underlying purpose in these investigations, their designs, methodologies, and measurement methods were evaluated using the four types of validity described by Cook and Campbell (1979): construct, internal, statistical conclusion, and external.

Construct Validity

Construct validity refers to the generalizability of one operation or measurement to a referent construct (Cook & Campbell, 1979). Construct validity applies not only to quasi-experimental, but also to descriptive research. Several problems concerning construct validity have been alluded to in previous sections of this chapter. Two threats to construct validity, however, deserve emphasis due to the magnitude of the problems encountered in nursing research on stress.

The first of the major threats to construct validity is called "inadequate preoperational explication of constructs" (Cook & Campbell, 1979, p. 64). The phenomenon refers to an imprecise definition of the construct under study that leads to the development of imprecise operationalizations and manipulations. The threat was present in over half of the studies reviewed (e.g., Beard, 1982; Volicer & Burns, 1977), and therefore appears to be a major stumbling block in development of meaningful nursing research regarding stress.

Two examples from studies reviewed are illustrative of inadequate preoperational explication of constructs. Nolan (1977) investigated the effect of quality of nursing care on stress of sedated surgical patients in a convenience sample of 100. Each of two groups received either routine care or actions to reduce stress. The dependent variable, stress, was defined as a response, yet measured by patient recall of the effects of interventions through use of a 12-item structured interview. From the researcher's description of the tool, it was unclear whether stress as a response was the actual dependent variable measured or whether the structured interview was tapping the subjects' perception of stressors. Nolan went on to state that "construct validity of the tool is claimed by the fact that the hypothesis was supported by the data collected" (p. 45). Such a conclusion clouds the issue of construct validity.

Another example of inadequate preoperational explication of stress was evident in a study by Hegedus (1979), in which 160 medical patients on four units received either primary or functional nursing care. While the investigator defined stress as considerable life adjustments following stressful events, a response-based construct, it was measured using the Volicer (1974) Hospital Stress Rating Scale, a stimulus-based scale.

Use of operational definitions or measurements that were not compatible with the conceptual definitions or theoretical framework of the study was a common problem and also is exemplified in the study conducted by Bell (1977). Bell identified the response model as the theoretical framework, but used the stimulus model tool developed by Holmes and Rahe (1967) to measure stress. Another example was the work of Foster (1974), in which a transactional theory base was identified and the presence of stress was inferred from Na/K ratios. In yet another example, Scott et al. (1984) identified a transactional theory base, yet they measured stress using the stimulus-based SRRS (Holmes & Rahe, 1967).

Other examples of definitional problems included: Miller and Grim (1979) defining stress as emotional stress, as a mood of feeling, and as concrete thinking; Schwartz & Brenner (1979) defining stress as additive, nonspecific physical effects, expectations of hospitalization, new stimuli, perception of hospital experience, and sensory deprivation; and Wert (1979) defining stress as symptoms produced by stressors. Such definitional ambiguity, together with incongruity between theoretical orientation and operationalization, suggested that a theoretical framework was often identified for conventional reasons rather than for the purpose of contributing to theory development through theory testing.

Careful attention to adequate preoperational explication of constructs would improve the quality of practice-relevant stress research. Padilla et al. (1981) and Sime (1976) demonstrated careful attention to construct definition and to the development of operationalizations clearly representative of the constructs. Padilla et al. carefully defined four types of information that lead to clear operationalization of four types of information given to patients prior to nasogastric intubation. Sime clearly defined preoperative fear, which led to the development of an unequivocal operational definition.

Confounding of variables was the second largest problem. The threat was present when various levels of treatment were not separated or when all possible levels of dependent variables or descriptive variables were not measured. For example, in a study reported by Brockway, Plummer, and Lowe (1976), the independent variable, type of reassurance, may have been confounded by the introduction of a tape recorder that was used to measure vocal stress.

Another example of confounding of variables was the presence of an unrecognized variable that mediates the effect of an independent variable. The existence of psychological stress often is inferred from physiological indices such as heart rate, blood pressure, Na/K ratios,

17-ketosteroids, and galvanic skin response (Errico, 1977; Foster, 1974; Guzzetta & Forsyth, 1979; Randolph, 1984). Psychological stress has also been inferred from the modulation of voice frequencies (Hurley, 1983). Evidence has suggested that such measures do not correspond well to psychological experiences, in part, because cognitive processes such as "attention" mediate physiological correlates (Appley & Trumbull, 1967; Mason, 1971, 1975a, 1975b). Although there was evidence to suggest that certain cognitive phenomena such as "uncertainty" triggered the release of corticosteroids and catecholamines (Warburton, 1979), it was a leap of faith to assume the presence or absence of "stress" from the aforementioned indices.

Manipulation checks can be utilized to determine whether or not an independent variable was operating in the expected manner (Wetzel, 1977). Several studies could have been improved with the use of manipulation checks, for example, the study by Brockway (1979) where the independent variable was the type of reassurance and the Ziemer (1983) study where the independent variable was type of information. In both studies it would have been helpful to ascertain whether or not treatment conditions actually were perceived by subjects as they were intended. Padilla et al. (1981) and Sime (1976) employed excellent manipulation checks and provided instructive examples of methods for improving construct validation.

Internal Validity

Internal validity is the second type of validity identified by Cook and Campbell (1979). Internal validity refers to support that a causal relationship is present and determination of the direction of that relationship. Threats to internal validity have been detailed in depth elsewhere (Cook & Campbell, 1979; Kerlinger, 1973).

Of all possible threats to internal validity, selection and history are the most troublesome in those studies reviewed. Selection, the most common problem, refers to the failure to account for inherent differences among groups studied. The threat occurs frequently in quasi-experimental research, where natural groupings of individuals receive differing treatments without random assignment to ensure quality. Several studies (Brockway et al., 1976; M. Johnson, 1979) reviewed would have benefited greatly by the random assignment of treatments to subjects.

History refers to the possibility that an observed effect may be due to systematic influences of events other than the treatment that occur between pre- and post-measures. In quasi-experimental research, particularly with hospitalized patients, efforts must be made to control for other variables that may interfere. In particular, the use of a control group or, when there is no control group, the use of a time series design would help to tease out the effects of history as a rival hypothesis. Attention to historical events was rarely mentioned in studies focused on patients receiving different treatments.

Statistical Conclusion Validity

Statistical conclusion validity is "valid inference-making" (Cook & Campbell, 1979, p. 37) based on statistical evidence. Three criteria must be met to claim statistical conclusion validity. The first is sensitivity represented by statistical power. Most researchers have not mentioned statistical power and have not used samples large enough to detect effects based on expected variances and levels of confidence. The danger here is that the likelihood of finding no significant difference when one is present increases when sample sizes are small and alpha levels are low (Cook & Campbell, 1979). Several studies (Brockway, 1979; Brockway et al., 1976; Foster, 1974; Minckley, 1974; Schwartz & Brenner, 1979) may have benefited by attention to statistical power. In a few cases, (Miller & Grim, 1979; Padilla et al., 1981), researchers reported trends based on alpha levels of .10. Such results may have actually represented differences that were obscured by small sample sizes.

Two additional statistical conclusion validity issues included reliability of measurement and random irrelevancies (Cook & Campbell, 1979). Several researchers reported reliabilities obtained in populations different from those with whom tools were currently being used, or made no mention of populations in which reliabilities were ascertained (Brandt, 1984; Murphy, 1984; Tilden, 1983). Occasional studies, however, did show concern for reliability estimates in the populations at hand (Smyth, Call, Hansell, Sparacino, & Strodtbeck, 1978; Volicer & Burns, 1977).

Random irrelevancies refer to extraneous sources of variance that differ across subjects (Cook & Campbell, 1979). Stress investigations in natural settings are replete with variables extraneous to those measured. In addition, it is difficult to force subjects' attention on the treatment at hand when other stressful aspects of experiences are also salient for subjects (Brockway et al., 1976; Volicer & Volicer, 1977). Random irrelevancies, however, deserve attention if research findings are to lead to predictively successful innovations in practice for the reduction of stress.

In general, problems with validity were present in over half of the studies reviewed. Problems most frequently noted were those concerning small sample sizes associated with problems of power and lack of evidence of reliability of measurement in the particular population investigated.

External Validity

External validity refers to the generalizability of findings across populations, settings, and times (Cook & Campbell, 1979). External validity, therefore is a requisite for the interpretation of results from all types of investigations, both quasi-experimental and descriptive, whether they utilize basic or applied approaches (Bickman, 1981).

The major external validity problem encountered was the use of nonrandomly selected samples. Approximately 90% of the investigations evaluated employed convenience sampling methods. Such a prevalent use of convenience sampling is a reflection of the difficulty in obtaining random samples in clinical research. A few investigators (e.g., Foster, 1974; Randolph, 1984; Ziemer, 1983) did use random assignment to improve the interpretation from convenience samples. In addition to use of random assignment when appropriate, the replication of studies using convenience sampling would greatly improve external validity.

While most researchers were mindful of not generalizing beyond their particular convenience sample, a few did imply generalizability beyond the constraints of the sample studied. Rarely were studies designed so that the researcher could generalize across time.

SUMMARY

Clearly, there is not agreement among nurse researchers regarding a definitional orientation to stress that best fits nursing's orientation to human experiences. Varying theoretical orientations are used to explain stress or stress-related phenomena, for example, stress as a stimulus, stress as a response, and stress as a transaction. The studies are fairly evenly distributed among the four definitional categories. The various approaches do not represent expanding theoretical explanations of stress, but rather are incompatible approaches to explaining stress.

More disconcerting than the lack of direction in research efforts, however, is that all too commonly the measurement of the variables and the methodology were not "linked" or consistent with the theoretical framework. For the most part the research efforts reviewed fell short of theory testing. Even for those studies that were designed to contribute to theory development, it was rare to find research reports that included implications regarding theory in the discussion sections. Additionally, discussion sections of the reports typically did not identify alternative explanations for the findings.

Quasi-experimental, ex post facto, and causal comparative studies typically were flawed with validity problems. If nursing is to strengthen its contribution to knowledge in the area of stress, more emphasis will need to be placed on congruence between design and measurement, and on issues of statistical rigor, validity, and reliability.

Although some might argue that it is too early to expect a coalescing of definitional orientations, it is important to point out that considerable confusion regarding stress phenomena results from a nonsystematic or nondeliberative mixture of incompatible orientations to or definitions of stress. It is little wonder that the vast number of opinion articles that appear in the nursing literature include varied definitions of stress, often making conflicting recommendations regarding the nursing assessment of stress and nursing intervention strategies to assist a person in stress management efforts.

RECOMMENDATIONS FOR
FUTURE RESEARCH

Nursing research about stress suffers from many of the same problems that plague stress research efforts in other disciplines. However, many of the serious theoretical, measurement, and methodological problems identified in our review are correctable. The following are recommendations for future research.

It is imperative that the researcher conceptually define all variables under study. Careful attention should be paid to developing operational definitions that are consistent with the theoretical orientation and conceptual definitions of constructs.

To ensure the integrity of the abstract concepts when operationalized, it is essential that strategies be employed to differentiate more clearly between and among constructs as well as measurement methods. One possible quantitative approach is the multitrait–multimethod matrix (Campbell & Fiske, 1959) used to define and describe convergent and divergent validity of concepts. Perhaps this method could be applied to studies such as the investigation by M. Johnson (1979) in which more than one closely related construct is apparent, such as anxiety and stress.

Greater emphasis should be placed on the discussion section of research reports. Particular attention should be paid to discussing the findings in relation to the theoretical base of the study (e.g., Scott, 1983) and by identifying possible alternative explanations of the findings.

Several suggestions for the improvement of validity deserve attention. Of particular importance is the attention to the issue of statistical power. There are three ways to increase statistical power: (a) increasing sample size; (b) increasing the effect size by increasing the frequency or intensity of the treatment; and (c) decreasing variance through increasing homogeneity of subjects or controlling for threats to internal validity (Cohen, 1977). Addressing the issue of statistical power may serve to clarify interpretation of otherwise inconclusive evidence regarding nursing interventions.

To improve internal validity, instruments should be assessed for stability (when measuring a construct that is proposed to be stable) and internal consistency. Not addressing internal consistency is problematic, particularly when using instruments with populations different from those in which reliability was established. Further improvement in internal validity could be accomplished through control of threats, such as history, to internal validity. Additionally, the use of manipulation checks would help to ensure that treatments are experienced by subjects in the way(s) proposed by the investigator.

To improve the generalizability of findings it is suggested that random samples be utilized whenever possible. When random sampling is not practical, subjects should be assigned randomly (e.g., Barsevick & Llewellyn, 1982) to treatment groups. The suggestion is forwarded with the knowledge that often external validity is enhanced to the detriment of internal validity.

A timely approach to practice-relevant stress research in nursing is the use of qualitative research to describe clearly how stress phenomena are experienced. Owing to the many problems with explication and operationalization of stress, it would seem wise to put more emphasis on descriptive and qualitative research. Efforts directed at defining complex stress phenomena should take first priority to help identify what people actually experience as stress.

Another viable approach to the study of stress is the investigation of intervening variables related to personal stress, for example, attention to behavioral rigidity (Schaie, 1955), relationships with significant others (Shaw, 1979), coping abilities and responses (House, 1981), and vulnerability (Kessler, 1979). The investigation of phenomena that mediate stress experiences would facilitate conceptualizations of stress that more accurately reflect life experience.

Current problems in stress research such as the difficulty in obtaining large sample sizes, difficulty in obtaining random samples, and the rival hypotheses prevalent in clinical research, support the need for replication of studies. Additionally, it is suggested here that nurse researchers interested in stress develop a program of research in a specific area.

In the preceding paragraphs we have emphasized areas of stress research needing improvement. The authors acknowledge that some fine studies, well conceived and executed, have been accomplished in the important area of stress research. However, the vast majority of studies reviewed had common and serious theoretical, methodological, and measurement flaws. It is hoped that the highlighting of such important and pervasive flaws will facilitate the design of investigations that have the potential for contributing to the body of nursing knowledge regarding stress.

REFERENCES

Anderson, M. D., & Pleticha, J. M. (1974). Emergency unit patients' perceptions of stressful life events. *Nursing Research, 23,* 378–383.

Appley, M. H., & Trumbull, R. (1967). *Psychological stress: Issues in research.* New York: Appleton-Century-Crofts.

Ballard, K. S. (1981). Identification of environmental stressors for patients in a surgical intensive care unit. *Issues in Mental Health Nursing, 3*(3), 89–108.

Barsevick, A., & Llewellyn, J. (1982). A comparison of the anxiety-reducing potential of two techniques of bathing. *Nursing Research, 31*, 22–27.

Beard, M. T. (1982). Trust, life events, and risk factors among adults. *Advances in Nursing Science, 4*(4), 26–43.

Bedsworth, J. A., & Molen, M. T. (1982). Psychological stress in spouses of patients with myocardial infarction. *Heart & Lung, 11*, 450–456.

Bell, J. M. (1977). Stressful life events and coping methods in mental-illness and -wellness behaviors. *Nursing Research, 26*, 136–141.

Bickman, L. (1981). Some distinctions between basic and applied approaches. *Applied Social Psychology Annual, 2*, 46–55.

Brandt, P. A. (1984). Stress-buffering effects of social support on maternal discipline. *Nursing Research, 33*, 229–234.

Brockway, B. F. (1979). Situational stress and temporal changes in self-report and vocal measurements. *Nursing Research, 28*, 20–24.

Brockway, B. F., Plummer, O. B., & Lowe, B. M. (1976). Effect of nursing reassurance on patient vocal stress levels. *Nursing Research, 25*, 440–446.

Campbell, D. T., & Fiske, E. W. (1959). Convergent and discriminant validation by the multitrait–multimethod matrix. *Psychological Bulletin, 56*, 81–105.

Cohen, J. (1977). *Statistical power analysis for the behavioral sciences.* New York: Academic Press.

Cook, T. D., & Campbell, D. T. (1979). *Quasi-experimental design and analysis: Issues in field settings.* Chicago: Rand McNally.

Errico, E. (1977). Effect of cardiac monitoring on blood pressure, apical rate and respiration with and without information feedback. *International Journal of Nursing Studies, 14*, 77–90.

Farr, L., Keene, A., Samson, D., & Michael, A. (1984). Alterations in circadian excretion of urinary variables and physiological indicators of stress following surgery. *Nursing Research, 33*, 140–146.

Foster, S. B. (1974). An adrenal measure for evaluating nursing effectiveness. *Nursing Research, 23*, 118–124.

Fuller, B. F., & Foster, G. M. (1982). The effects of family/friend visits vs. staff interaction on stress/arousal of surgical intensive care patients. *Heart & Lung, 11*, 457–463.

Guzzetta, C. E. (1979). Relationship between stress and learning. *Advances in Nursing Science, 1*(4), 35–49.

Guzzetta, C. E., & Forsyth, G. L. (1979). Nursing diagnostic pilot study: Psychophysiologic stress. *Advances in Nursing Science, 2*(1), 27–44.

Hardy, M. E. (1974). Theories: Components, development, and evaluation. *Nursing Research, 23*, 100–106.

Haughey, B. P., Brasure, J., Maloney, M. M., & Graham, S. (1984). The relationship between stressful life events and electrocardiogram abnormalities. *Heart & Lung, 13*, 405–410.

Hegedus, K. S. (1979). A patient outcome criterion measure . . . Volicer Hospital Stress Rating Scale. *Supervisor Nurse, 10*(1), 40–45.

Hoffman, M., Donckers, S., & Hauser, M. (1978). The effect of nursing intervention on stress factors perceived by patients coronary care units. *Heart & Lung, 7*, 804–809.

Holmes, T. H., & Masuda, M. (1966). Magnitude estimations of social readjustments. *Journal of Psychosomatic Research, 11*, 219–225.

Holmes, T. H., & Rahe, R. (1967). The social readjustment rating scale. *Journal of Psychosomatic Research, 12*, 213–218.

House, J. S. (1981). *Work stress and social support*. Reading, MA: Addison-Wesley.

Hurley, P. M. (1983). Communication variables and voice analysis of marital conflict stress. *Nursing Research, 32*, 164–169.

Jalowiec, A., & Powers, M. J. (1981). Stress and coping in hypertensive and emergency room patients. *Nursing Research, 30*, 10–14.

Johnson, J. E. (1984). Coping with elective surgery. In H. H. Werley & J. J. Fitzpatrick (Eds.), *Annual Review of Nursing Research* (Vol. 2) (pp. 107–132). New York: Springer Publishing.

Johnson, J. H., & Sarason, I. G. (1979). Recent developments in research on life stress. In V. Hamilton & D. M. Warburton (Eds.), *Human stress and cognition: An information processing approach* (pp. 205–233). London: Wiley.

Johnson, M. (1979). Anxiety/stress and the effects on disclosure between nurses and patients. *Advances in Nursing Science, 1*(4), 1–20.

Kerlinger, F. N. (1973). *Foundations of behavioral research* (2nd ed.). New York: Holt, Rinehart, & Winston.

Kessler, R. C. (1979). A strategy for studying differential vulnerability to the psychological consequence of stress. *Journal of Health and Social Behavior, 20*, 100–108.

Kobasa, S. C. (1979). Stessful life events, personality, and health: An inquiry into hardiness. *Journal of Personality and Social Psychology, 37*, 1–11.

Kobasa, S. C., Maddi, S. R., & Kan, S. (1982). Hardiness and health: A prospective study. *Journal of Personality and Social Psychology, 42*, 168–177.

Lazarus, R. S. (1966). *Psychological stress and the coping process*. New York: McGraw-Hill.

Mason, J. W. (1971). A re-evaluation of the concept of "non-specificity" in stress theory. *Journal of Psychiatric Research, 8*, 323–333.

Mason, J. W. (1975a). A historical view of the stress field: Part I. *Journal of Human Stress, 1*, 6–12.

Mason, J. W. (1975b). A historical view of the stress field: Part II. *Journal of Human Stress, 1*, 22–36.

Miller, C., & Grim, C. (1979). Personality and emotional stress measurement on hypertensive patients with essential and secondary hypertension. *International Journal of Nursing Studies, 16*, 83–93.

Minckley, B. B. (1974). Physiologic and psychologic responses of elective surgical patients. *Nursing Research, 23*, 392–401.

Mishel. M. H. (1984). Perceived uncertainty and stress in illness. *Research in Nursing and Health, 7*, 163–171.

Murphy, S. (1984). Stress levels and health status of victims of a natural disaster. *Research in Nursing and Health, 7*, 205–215.

Nolan, M. R. (1977). Effects of nursing intervention in the operating room as recalled on the third postoperative day. In M. V. Batey (Ed.), *Communicating nursing research*, (Vol. 9) (pp. 41–50). Boulder, CO: Western Interstate Commission for Higher Education.

Norbeck, J. S. (1984). Modification of life event questionnaires for use with female respondents. *Research in Nursing and Health, 7*, 61–71.

Padilla, G. P., Grant, M. M., Rains, B. L., Hansen, B. C., Bergstrom, N., Wong, H. L., Hanson R., & Kubo, W. (1981). Distress reduction and the effects of preparatory teaching films and patient control. *Research in Nursing and Health, 4*, 375–387.

Rahe, R. H. (1977). Life change measurement clarification. *Psychosomatic Medicine*, *40*, 95–98.

Randolph, G. L. (1984). Therapeutic and physical touch: Physiological response to stressful stimuli. *Nursing Research*, *33*, 33–36.

Sarason, I. G., Johnson, J. H., & Siegel, J. M. (1978). Assessing the impact of life changes: Development of the Life Experiences Survey. *Journal of Consulting and Clinical Psychology*, *46*, 932–946.

Schaie, K. W. (1955). A test of behavior rigidity. *Journal of Abnormal Psychology*, *51*, 604–608.

Schwartz, L. P., & Brenner, Z. R.(1979). Critical care unit transfer: Reducing patient stress through nursing interventions. *Heart & Lung*, *8*, 540–546.

Scott, D. W. (1983). Anxiety, critical thinking and information processing during and after breast biopsy. *Nursing Research*, *32*, 24–34.

Scott, D. W., Oberst, M. T., & Bookbinder, M. I. (1984). Stress–coping response to genitourinary carcinoma in men. *Nursing Research*, *33*, 325–329.

Selye, H. (1956). *The stress of life*. New York: McGraw-Hill.

Selye, H. (1976). *The stress of life*. (2nd Ed.). New York: McGraw-Hill.

Shaw, E. E. (1979). Health education for the public: Stress and stress management. *Topics in Clinical Nursing*, *1*(1), 53–57.

Sime, M. (1976). Relationship of preoperative fear, type of coping, and information received about surgery to recovery from surgery. *Journal of Personality and Social Psychology*, *34*, 716–724.

Smyth, K., Call, J. Hansell, S., Sparacino, J., & Strodtbeck, F. (1978). Type A behavior pattern and hypertension among inner-city black women. *Nursing Research*, *27*, 30–35.

Stember, M. L. (1977). Familial response to hospitalization of an adult family member. In M. V. Batey (Ed.), *Communicating nursing research* (Vol. 9) (pp. 59–75). Boulder, CO: Western Interstate Commission for Higher Education.

Tamez, E., Moore, M., & Brown, P. (1978). Relaxation training as a nursing intervention versus pro re nata medication. *Nursing Research*, *27*, 160–165.

Tilden, V. P. (1983). The relation of life stress and social support to emotional disequilibrium during pregnancy. *Research in Nursing and Health*, *6*, 167–174.

Toth, J. C. (1980). Effect of structure preparation for transfer on patient anxiety on leaving coronary care unit. *Nursing Research*, *29*, 28–34.

Volicer, B. J. (1974). Patient's perceptions of stressful events associated with hospitalization. *Nursing Research*, *23*, 235–238.

Volicer, B. J. (1977). Stress factors in the experience of hospitalization. In M. V. Batey (Ed.), *Communicating nursing research*, (Vol. 8) (pp. 53–67). Boulder, CO: Western Interstate Commission for Higher Education.

Volicer, B. J., & Bohannon, M. W. (1975). A hospital stress rating scale. *Nursing Research*, *24*, 352–359.

Volicer, B. J., & Burns, M. W. (1977). Preexisting correlates of hospital stress. *Nursing Research*, *26*, 408–415.

Volicer, B. J., & Volicer, L. (1977). Cardiovascular changes associated with stress during hospitalization. *Journal of Psychosomatic Research*, *22*, 159–168.

Walker, K. L., & Avant, K. D. (1983). *Strategies for theory construction in nursing*. Norwalk, CT: Appleton-Century Crofts.

Warburton, D. M. (1979). Physiological aspects of information processing and stress. In V. Hamilton & D. M. Warburton (Eds.), *Human stress and cogni-*

tion: An information processing approach (pp. 33–65). New York: Wiley.
Wert, B. J. (1979). Stress due to nuclear accident: A survey of an employee population. *Occupational Health Nursing, 27*(9), 16–24.
Wetzel, C. G. (1977). Manipulation checks: A reply to Kid. *Representative Research in Social Psychology, 8*, 88–93.
Ziemer, M. M. (1983). Effects of information on postsurgical coping. *Nursing Research, 32*, 282–287.

Chapter 2

Pain

ANN GILL TAYLOR
SCHOOL OF NURSING
UNIVERSITY OF VIRGINIA

CONTENTS

Research on pain has received extensive multidisciplinary attention over the last two decades. Because of this attention, nurses have increased their theoretical understanding of and contributions to pain research. Based on these contributions, the purpose of this review is to delineate and critique substantive areas of pain research in nursing and to infer generalizations about issues represented in the research.

This review of pain research in nursing covered the period 1961 through 1984, a period that coincides with the early development of nursing research on the topic of pain. In addition, four 1985 publications were included that were significant contributions to the nursing

The author gratefully acknowledges the contributions of Linda Little, doctoral candidate, Beth Rodgers, doctoral student, and Sister Lisa Marie Drover, master's student, who played important roles in screening and retrieving the research articles. In addition, the author acknowledges the reference librarians of the University of Virginia Claude Moore Health Sciences Library, and School of Nursing secretaries Janice Martin, Debra Peters, and Gwen Christmas, who carefully typed the many revisions of the manuscript.

23

literature. To locate nursing research on pain, the following retrieval strategies were used: (a) computer searches using MEDLINE and PsychINFO data bases, (b) manual searches of the *Cumulative Index to Nursing and Allied Health Literature*, and (c) review of the *Directory of Nurses with Doctoral Degrees, 1984*, as well as a review of awards from the American Nurses' Foundation and Sigma Theta Tau to locate nurses who identified pain as a research interest.

The criteria for selecting a publication for inclusion in the review were that it was a report of research published between 1961 and 1984 and included a clearly stated research question, evidence of systematic data collection, analysis of data, and stated conclusions. Because of space constraints, the review was representative rather than exhaustive and did not include unpublished pain studies such as dissertations or master's theses. The specialized field of pediatric pain was not included.

Several authors have published reviews of pain research. Anderson (1982), Kim (1980), and Peric-Knowlton (1984) have conducted pain study reviews with a distinct focus. Anderson (1982) presented an overview of literature on pain interventions for cancer patients. She concluded from the research on nursing practice that a consistent approach to the assessment of the cancer patient experiencing pain has been lacking and development of assessment tools is needed. Anderson noted the need for nurses to monitor their knowledge and practice continually because fear of patient addiction and a reactive rather than proactive approach to dosage intervals were common attitudes held among both physicians and nurses.

Kim (1980) reviewed pain theory, research, and nursing practice with an eye to building nursing theory related to pain care and to the formulation of effective planned nursing interventions in the clinical setting. The review included research findings on the relationship between pain and patient characteristics and on interventions such as information and attention. She provided an excellent critique of reliability and validity problems in the research, and offered a list of recommendations for future studies.

Peric-Knowlton (1984) reviewed current trends in nursing practice related to the care of the adult patient with acute pain and provided an excellent discussion of contemporary pain theories; she addressed the effects of nursing interaction, preoperative teaching, and nonpharmacologic, noninvasive pain relief methods. A list of substantive suggestions for better implementation of existing research findings was presented.

In two recent reviews Beyer and Byers (1985) and Eland (1985) offered representative treatment of nursing research in the specialized area of pediatric pain. Eland's chapter dealt principally with assessment issues and problems, and she cited the instruments that have been developed for assessment in children's pain. Beyer and Byers' review of research on pediatric pain was organized into four areas of concern: consequences of pain, pain assessment, the pain experience, and management of pain. Various assessment approaches were discussed fully. In the reviews by Eland and Beyer and Byers, and elsewhere (e.g., Beyer, DeGood, Ashley, & Russell, 1983; Eland & Anderson, 1977), concern was expressed about the differences in analgesic administration for children's and adults' pain, considering the lack of conclusive evidence that children need less analgesics. More collaborative work is needed with researchers in fields such as child psychology in order to understand better how children experience pain and the long-term effects that early pain experiences may have. Abu-Saad (1984) had further work underway to examine how well physiological and behavioral scales are correlated with school-age children's verbalization of pain.

In the first part of the present review, factors influencing assessment of pain are addressed, whereas in the second part of the review the management of pain is addressed. Major concepts and themes in the studies were used as the organizing framework for the review; the studies are grouped conceptually within the organizing framework. The questions that guided the review were: (a) What are the major findings within the substantive areas of the research? (b) To what populations are the findings limited? (c) What major conceptual or methodological strengths and limitations exist? and (d) What do the studies contribute to nursing knowledge about pain assessment and management?

FACTORS INFLUENCING ASSESSMENT OF PAIN

Measurement Tools

The problem of measurement has been particularly difficult for the pain researcher. Thus, a significant portion of work in pain has gone into the development of objective measures of pain that can be used in the clinical setting. An example of such studies was conducted by Geden, Beck, Brouder, and O'Connell (1983), who measured correlational relationships among four laboratory stimuli: modified submaximum effort tourniquet technique, Forgione-Barber pain stimulator, cold water stimulus and faradic shock, and contraction ratings of 40 primiparous women. Using the McGill Pain Questionnaire (Melzack, 1975), the contractions were rated 24 to 48 hours after delivery whereas the laboratory stimuli were rated 6 to 8 weeks postpartum. They concluded that in order to serve as a realistic analogue of labor contractions during the transitional phase, a laboratory pain stimulus needed to be delivered for periods of approximately 80 seconds with 75-second interstimulus intervals. Although these researchers improved upon the methodological shortcomings of earlier analogue research on labor pain, they concluded that there was no guarantee that their laboratory findings would generalize to the real-world practice settings.

Burckhardt (1984) carried out a principal components analysis of the responses to the McGill Pain Questionnaire to determine its appropriateness for describing the unique type of pain experienced by arthritis patients. Only one factor accounted for any significant amount (29%) of the variance. The factor was weighted heavily by the affective subclasses, suggesting a significant affective–reactive component of arthritis pain that needed further study. The work of Stewart (1977) in developing a Pain-Color Scale and Pain Circles represented yet another approach to pain measurement and showed promise for assessing the qualitative aspects of the pain experience.

A useful reference has been prepared by McGuire (1984), who reviewed the instruments that have been developed for use in the clinical assessment and management of pain. She classified the instruments according to the pain dimension(s) being measured, instrument reliability and validity, type of pain for which best suited, and requirements for administration.

General Pain Indices

Several studies have been conducted to describe general indices used by nurses to assess pain. Studies conducted in nonclinical settings, using either vignettes or descriptive statements of patients, show conflicting results. Baer, L. Davitz, and Lieb (1970) reported that nurses inferred more pain from verbal than nonverbal communication, and

Jacox and Stewart (1973) and Oberst (1978) reported more pain inferred from nonverbal communication. In the clinical setting, nurses reported that physiological signs and behaviors were easier indexes to use in pain assessment than verbal report (Jacox, 1979), yet data from oncology nurses' notes (Bagley, Falinski, Garnizo, & Hooker, 1982) indicated that administration of pain relieving medication was based mostly on cancer patient's verbalization of their pain. Investigators for the latter studies did not take into account whether congruence existed between nurses' notes and the actual decision-making process.

Teske, Daut, and Cleeland (1983) used standardized observational ratings of medical-surgical patients and pain clinic outpatients to examine the relationship between patients' self-report of pain and nurses' inferences based on nonverbal behavior. They found agreement among nurses to be high when judging pain, but a low correspondence between nurses' judgments of pain and patients' self-report of pain. Teske et al.'s results were consistent with findings from Graffam's earlier survey (1981) of hospitalized medical-surgical patients, 75% of whom had chronic pain. Although her data analyses were not described adequately, Graffam reported congruence in nurse–patient expectations regarding the occurrence and severity of pain, but significant disparity in nurse–patient ratings of severe pain. Where there was disagreement, 80% or more of the patients judged the pain to be more severe than did the nurses.

In an early study, Hammond, Kelly, Schneider, and Vancini (1966) explored the tasks involved in pain assessment following abdominal surgery. They concluded that nurses were confronted by a very large number of cognitive tasks in relieving pain, and that none of the characteristics of the tasks analyzed could be the basis for specific nursing actions. A decade later Oberst (1978) expressed a pressing need for systematic conceptualization of the pain assessment process because of preconceived notions about pain that impeded nurses' accurate and sensitive pain assessment.

To summarize, review of the research describing general indices used by nurses in assessing pain suggests that (a) nurses' pain assessments are not standardized, which has caused some investigators to temper interpretations of their results with comments about the limitations of the measurement techniques; (b) nurses use some combination of observable pain behaviors and verbal expression as pain indices; and (c) nurses' assessments are not necessarily congruent with patients' pain needs.

Nurses' Inferences

Research findings on nurses' inferences of psychological distress associated with pain have indicated that nurses consistently rated psychological distress associated with pain higher than physical suffering (Dudley & Holm, 1984; Lenburg, Glass, & Davitz, L., 1970) and that nurses inferred greater psychological distress from patients' nonverbal actions than from their verbal communication (Baer et al., 1970). A number of researchers have examined variables that may have accounted for patterns of nurses' inferences. Overall, no relationship has been found between nurses' inferences and professional characteristics such as educational preparation, clinical specialty, job satisfaction, and employment position (Dudley & Holm, 1984; Mason, 1981). Virtually all studies of the relationship of professional nursing characteristics to inferences have been conducted using hospital-based nurses. The profession would benefit from study of nurses in other settings. Mason (1981) did find differences in inferences of physical suffering related to years in practice: nurses with the lesser amount of experience inferred the greatest degree of physical suffering. Dudley and Holm (1984), however, did not find any relationship between years of practice and inferences of suffering as measured by the Standard Measure of Inferences of Suffering.

In studies of personal characteristics of the nurse, age was not a significant factor influencing inferences, whereas the patient's age has been a significant factor across the majority of studies where it was included as a variable (Davitz, L., Davitz, J., & Higuchi, 1977a, 1977b; Davitz, L. & Pendleton, 1969; Mason, 1981; Taylor, Skelton, & Butcher, 1984). Other major nurse or patient characteristics related to nurses' inferences were cultural or ethnic background and perceived socioeconomic background (Baer, Davitz, L., & Lieb, 1970; Davitz, L. & Davitz, J., 1975; Davitz, L. L. et al., 1977a, 1977b; Davitz, L. & Pendleton, 1969; Lenburg, Burnside, & Davitz, L., 1970; Lenburg, Glass, & Davitz, L., 1970). The recent (1981) L. Davitz and J. Davitz book, *Inferences of Patients' Pain and Psychological Distress: Studies of Nursing Behaviors* was a classic presentation of research on the relationship between characteristics and belief systems and nursing behavior in pain assessment and management.

Aside from nurses' characteristics, variables associated with the pain condition such as diagnosis, physical pathology, and duration of the pain condition have been associated with nurses' inferences of suffering (Dudley & Holm, 1984; Oberst, 1978; Taylor, Skelton, & Butcher, 1984). In addition, both Oberst and Taylor et al. reported greater inferences of pain if physical pathology was evident, suggesting lesser inferences for patients having chronic pain symptoms without evident physical pathology. Using patient vignettes, Taylor et al. also found that nurses' ratings of personality and behavioral traits were more negative for patients with low back pain than for those with headache or joint pain. Teske et al.'s (1983) finding of greater discrepancies between nurses' and patients' ratings of pain in a chronic pain sample than in an acute pain sample supports Oberst's and Taylor et al.'s findings. Because the Oberst and Taylor et al. studies were "paper-and-pencil" studies, replication is needed in clinical settings.

Several investigators have described nurses' pain assessment behavior, attitudes, or beliefs in an attempt to identify the factors influencing the pain assessment and management process. Cohen's (1980) interview data from postsurgical patients about their pain status and nurses' medication choices indicated that 75% of the patients were in moderate or marked pain and that a general question did not assess pain adequately. Chart review and nurses' questionnaire findings also indicated that patients were receiving less narcotic analgesics than they could have received, and that nurses were overly concerned about the possibility of addiction. Rankin and Snider's (1984) questionnaire data from oncology nurses indicated that the nurses found a moderate level of pain reduction adequate, except for patients suffering intense pain. Hunt, Stollar, Littlejohns, Twycross, and Vere (1977) had 13 patients with protracted pain assess their pain using visual analogues and found that few patients were free of pain as a result of nursing interventions. Likewise, Graffam (1970, 1981), using observational and questionnaire data, described nurse assessment of pain as minimal, documenting that nurses for the most part did not assess pain thoroughly and systematically. Pain relief measures typically were provided when the patient asked for them, and usually only the single relief measure of medication was provided. In sum, findings from these studies suggested a need for increased education among nurses about patients' pain behavior and its assessment and management.

Research on the organizational environment in which pain assessment and management occur was represented in only two studies. Strauss, Fagerhaugh, and Glaser (1974) made systematic observations on approximately 20 selected wards in nine hospitals for the purpose of grounding a new perspective on pain in the organizational settings in which pain management and patient care take place. They found that nurses had preconceived ideas and expectations about the degree of suffering associated with various diagnoses and prognoses, and seemed to have difficulty dealing with behaviors that deviated from the expected. They also concluded that substantial improvements in the care of patients in pain would prove difficult unless organizational features were taken into account. With the exception of Fagerhaugh's (1974) publication applying the framework to a burn care unit, no other research was located that built upon the Strauss, Fagerhaugh, and Glaser model. Those authors concluded that organizational features figured largely in the delivery of pain care and have conceptualized organizational dimensions through which the administration of pain care may be analyzed; but further study in this area is needed.

In summary, review of the research findings on factors influencing nurses' inference of pain suggests the need for (a) continued, upgraded study of factors that influence the assessment process and (b) development of models of appropriate assessment dimensions that nurses should consider in pain assessment.

MANAGEMENT OF PAIN

The topic of pain management was researched from two basic perspectives: (a) patient variables influencing pain management and (b) nursing interventions. Finally, a group of studies on comprehensive pain treatment programs was reviewed.

Patient Variables

Individual variability in responding to pain has been approached in several different ways. Copp (1974, 1985a, 1985b) has studied the experiences and feelings of patients who suffer from pain, and through a model and typology has provided qualitative description and classification of the different meanings that patients attach to the pain experience. Other researchers have investigated the relationship between patient variables and patients' pain responses. Walike and

Meyer (1966) explored the variables of ego strength and anxiety in relation to placebo responsivity for rheumatoid arthritis patients attending a medical clinic. Correlations were found that showed placebo reactors exhibited higher dependency and anxiety and lower ego strength and self-sufficiency than others in the sample. Although this early study tended to suggest negative connotations for placebo response, today the placebo effect is recognized as an important psychological component of treatment strategies.

Bruegel (1971) and Bradford (1981) measured the influence of anxiety upon pain. Bruegel reported no relationship between anxiety and postoperative pain perception, and Bradford did not find a significant relationship between anxiety and frequency of chest pain medications. Jacox and Stewart (1973) studied three patient groups classified according to short-term, long-term, and progressive pain to determine the relationships among the personality factors of neuroticism and extroversion, pain-related psychosocial problems reported by patients, and type of pain. No consistent relationship between neuroticism and pain intensity was found when types of pain associated with different conditions were considered. However, elevations in scores for neuroticism on standardized personality tests in pain patients have been reported in psychology studies (e.g., Engel, 1959; Sternbach, 1975; Watson, 1982). It seems the longer the patients have suffered, the more disturbed they have become as measured by these tests. However, it may have been that personality variables were simply different for people with different pain conditions. More work of the conceptual breadth exemplified by Jacox and Stewart is needed, building upon existing knowledge bases in nursing and related disciplines.

Age was the most significant factor influencing patient responsivity to drugs as measured by analgesic potency assays in cancer patients with chronic pain (Kaiko, Wallenstein, Rogers, Grabinski, & Houde, 1982). Plasma morphine levels were higher in older subjects, and the exponential rate of decline of plasma morphine was related significantly and inversely to the age of the patient.

Bradford (1981) studied marital adjustment as a patient factor related to pain in male postmyocardial infarction patients, using self-report instruments. She found that marital adjustment related negatively to chest pain: Men scoring higher on marital adjustment required less chest pain medication. Continued exploration of patient variables and the pain experience is needed.

Nursing Interventions

Nurse–Patient Interaction. Research on the effectiveness of nursing interventions for pain management constituted the majority of studies for this review. Diers, Schmidt, McBride, and Davis (1972) reviewed studies from the 1960s on the effectiveness on pain of varying levels of purposive interaction between nurses and patients. The cumulative evidence from these and later studies suggested that more interactive, attentive involvement by nurses in the management of patients' pain resulted in (a) reduced levels of patients' pain; (b) quicker pain relief; and (c) in some cases, reduced dependence upon medication as the sole treatment (Bochnak, 1982; McBride, 1966; Moss, 1967; Moss & Meyer, 1966). However, when Chambers and Price (1967) conducted an experimental study of 125 medical–surgical patients to determine whether positive or distracting statements by nurses at the time they gave an analgesic influenced the relief of pain, the results neither supported nor ruled out the use of nurses' statements. Jacox (1979) and others described components of pain that were more psychosocial than physical in nature, and Diers et al. and others reported evidence of the relief of distress, discomfort, and anxiety by interactive nursing interventions. However, the lack of consistent definition and operationalization of interactive nursing approaches used in the research was a persistent problem (Chambers & Price, 1967). Diers et al. (1972) addressed this problem in their study by using a categorization scheme of nursing approaches based on psychosomatic pain theory. The authors found that even with identical instructions for operationalization of the nursing approaches and category definitions, nurses implemented the approaches somewhat differently. No quasi-experimental or experimental research on the effectiveness of deliberative nurse–patient interaction was identified after 1972.

In a descriptive study of nursing practice in pain relief, Hunt et al. (1977) ascertained that nurses rarely used deliberative, interactive techniques in pain management. Additional study of nursing approaches should be conducted using appropriate theoretical bases and more tightly controlled operational conditions.

Patient Instruction or Information. Researchers have conducted a number of studies over the last two decades to examine preoperative instruction in coping strategies for pain reduction (Healy, 1968; Johnson, Rice, Fuller, & Endress, 1981; Voshall, 1980). Only tentative conclusions could be drawn from these studies because there was only approximate overlap in methods. However, preoperative instruction did have an effect upon the number of analgesics received, rate of recovery, and associated variables.

In a laboratory study, Mulcahy and Janz (1973) found that brief instruction on a combination of techniques significantly raised pain threshold means for subjects experiencing induced pain. Other laboratory-based research showed that distress levels associated with ischemic pain were reduced by relevant information on sensations to be experienced (Johnson, 1973; Johnson & Rice, 1974). However, congruent with the clinical research on preoperative instruction, pain intensity levels were not affected significantly. These studies supported earlier work indicating that pain thresholds varied as a function of instructions given subjects (Blitz & Dinnerstein, 1968), and the main reason seemed to be response bias, which has been worse when the stimulus produced nonnoxious sensation over a large range of intensities before it produced pain. A recent study by Manderino and Bzdek (1984) incorporated videotaping to test the effects of both modeling and information on the pain reactions of nulliparous female college students. The only significant reduction in pain ratings occurred for the combination of information and modeling via videotape.

Interventions to Relieve Pain of Injections.   A group of studies was conducted on intervention strategies to reduce pain associated with injections. Carter (1967) compared individual pain reactions to injections of distilled water and normal saline given to female student nurse volunteers. Both types of injections produced discomfort, but the distilled water produced greater discomfort. Perez (1984) reported that increasing the duration of injection time resulted in less pain intensity, as measured by a finger dynamometer pinch gauge. Position of limbs as a factor affecting pain intensity in injections was examined by Itty, Kurian, and Cherian (1977) using medical–surgical patients in a hospital setting. Subjects placed in the semi-prone position reported less injection pain for gluteal and deltoid muscle injections than subjects in the side-lying position. Levin (1982) studied choice of injection site and locus of control as patient variables influencing the perception of momentary pain and found no significant relationships.

Perhaps the analgesic drug effect achieved from a given injection site would be more important than the pain experienced with injections. Site of injection and type of analgesia were compared in an excellent exploratory study by Grabinski (1983). She reported more rapid and greater degree of pain relief from the use of the deltoid site over the gluteal site for methodane, whereas deltoid and gluteal injections of morphine produced comparable pain relief.

Relaxation. A number of investigators have focused on relaxation as an intervention for pain. For example, Cunningham (1974) found with six discolysis patients that the use of auditory biofeedback to induce muscle relaxation resulted in significantly reduced lower back pain, as measured by EMGs and patient self-report. A prior experiment by Cunningham suggested that it made no difference whether biofeedback or verbal instructions were given to teach muscle relaxation, and that specialized equipment may not have been necessary to achieve the same end result. Flaherty and Fitzpatrick (1978) studied postoperative elective surgery patients using a relaxation technique that focused on muscles associated with cognition and speech for an experimental group; the control group was not taught the technique. Mean differences in reports of incisional pain and body distress, analgesic consumption, and respiratory rate changes were statistically significant, supporting use of the relaxation technique. In a study of the effect of progressive relaxation training upon cancer patients, Kaempfer (1982) concluded that reduction of muscle tension not always would be a suitable stress management technique for this population, due to the concentration on body functions and sustained mental and physical effort required.

Graffam (1984) surveyed health care practitioners to ascertain their experience with untoward reactions to relaxation strategies and found a relative absence of untoward reactions. Graffam's work corroborated the findings of Cunningham (1974), Flaherty and Fitzpatrick (1978), and Horowitz, Fitzpatrick, and Flaherty (1984), which suggested that relaxation therapies may be considered a viable option in pain reduction.

Combined Cognitive-Behavioral Strategies. Various combinations of cognitive-behavioral strategies to reduce pain were the focus of five studies. Laborde and Powers (1983) conducted a study of patients suffering from chronic osteoarthritic joint pain, randomly assigning patients to a control group or to one of four treatment groups: (a) information brochure, (b) joint preservation teaching; (c) joint relaxation teaching plus brochure; and (d) joint preservation teaching, joint relaxation teaching, and brochure. Using a two-way analysis of variance, the authors reported a significant main effect for type of intervention. Subjects who received the relaxation procedure (c above) and the combined procedure (d above) reported significantly less pain on the Melzack Pain Intensity Rating Scale (Melzack, 1975) than subjects receiving the information brochure alone. Wells (1982), using a sample of 12 cholecystectomy patients with 6 in each treatment group, compared the effects of preoperative instruction and a structured relaxation program on abdominal muscle tension and pain intensity and distress ratings. Relaxation training did not alter abdominal muscle tension compared to the control group, but experimental subjects did report less psychological distress. The physical intensity of pain as measured by the Johnson (1973) pain rating scale was not significantly different between the groups.

Geden, Beck, Hauge, and Pohlman (1984) studied the effects of various combinations of cognitive-behavioral pain coping strategies during labor preparation analogues for 100 nulliparous female college students. Students were assigned to 1 of 10 treatment conditions: (a) pleasant imagery, (b) pleasant imagery plus relaxation training, (c) sensory transformation, (d) sensory transformation plus relaxation, (e) neutral imagery, (f) neutral imagery plus relaxation, (g) combined strategies, (h) combined strategies plus relaxation, (i) relaxation only, and (j) no treatment. Each of the 10 groups received a 1-hour training session, and 1 week later the subjects received 20 80-second exposures to the Forgione-Barber pain stimulator with 75-second interstimulus intervals. Examination of the treatment effect by the Newman-Keuls procedure showed that subjects in the sensory transformation group who were taught to transform the experience of the laboratory pain stimulus into a pleasant feeling performed significantly better across 20 trials than subjects receiving neutral imagery or those receiving no treatment. The other seven groups fell between the two groups and did not differ significantly from one another. Data analyses conducted on self-reported pain supported the authors' contention that certain treatment components, particularly sensory transformation, were more useful than others as pain-coping strategies. Geden et al. interpreted the unfavorable findings for the effects of pleasant imagery and the combination of pleasant imagery, sensory transformation, and neutral imagery as a function of the extensive stimulus exposure, compared to limited exposure in several other studies.

Two investigators examined interventions using rhythmic therapy—lightwaves and music—to provide distraction and relaxation in bringing about pain reduction in female subjects. Locsin (1981) investigated the effect of music on the pain of obstetric and gynecologic patients during the first 48 postoperative hours. Significant differences in values for musculoskeletal and verbal pain reactions were found between experimental and control groups. Subjects in the control group were not provided with their musical preference. McDonald (1982) studied the relationship between the human experience of pain and the use of colored light in the environment with volunteer rheumatoid arthritis outpatients. She found a relationship between light-wave length and duration (i.e., color) and patients' pain intensity, with the shorter, more frequent waves (blue) associated with greater reduction in pain. Additionally, the longer the exposure to lightwaves the greater was the likelihood of reduction in pain. In sum, findings in recent research on cognitive-behavioral nursing interventions to reduce pain have suggested that more positive results are achieved with interventions that engage both the senses and cognition.

Transcutaneous Electrical Nerve Stimulation. Another type of noninvasive intervention represented in the research was transcutaneous electrical nerve stimulation (TENS). Research on TENS historically has been done by physicians, with three recent studies by nurses who examined it as an alternative to narcotic analgesics for pain reduction (Dunbar, 1976; Moore & Blacker, 1983; Taylor, West, Simon, Skelton, & Rowlingson, 1983). Findings by Taylor et al. indicated that TENS may be effective in treating acute postoperative pain. They found that patient groups treated with TENS showed significantly more pain relief than patients treated with narcotics alone. Findings by Dunbar and Moore and Blacker suggested that TENS was markedly successful in relieving pain from postabdominal surgery, back pain, and specific kinds of neurosurgically related pain. However, in the case of headaches, other kinds of neurosurgically related pain, and miscellaneous types of pain, TENS was less successful.

Comprehensive Pain Treatment Programs. A final group of researchers addressed the intervention role of nurses by developing and field-testing comprehensive pain management programs, using various combinations of analgesic regimen and instruction about pain behavior and assessment (Degner, Fujii, & Levitt, 1982; Pierce & Ya Deau, 1980; Sofaer, 1983). Rankin (1982) studied pain of hospitalized cancer patients and reported that they continued to have moderate levels of pain and distress in spite of their analgesic regimens. As did Pierce and Ya Deau, Degner et al. stated that the most significant outcome of their study was the improved quality of life for patients with chronic pain; better pain control resulted from changes in staff attitudes and pain management practices. What distinguished the approaches of Pierce and Ya Deau, Degner et al., and Sofaer was their objective of controlling pain rather than simply responding to it. These studies of comprehensive pain relief programs have provided excellent models for future field-based research efforts toward pain treatment. However, consideration needs to be given to the incorporation of comparison groups.

CONCLUSIONS AND
RESEARCH DIRECTIONS

A major finding of this review was the need for more nursing research on pain. Although certain topics received more attention than others, allowing some accrual of findings, replication of studies was almost nonexistent. Of particular concern was the near absence of replication studies that extended the methodology of original studies by using improved controls and multiple treatment levels or conditions. Despite the progress that has been made during the past two decades, serious problems in measurement theory and methodology have remained that have impact on the quality of pain research in nursing as well as other fields. Difficulties existed in inferring pain from the various indirect measurement procedures that have been used. Assessment of patients experiencing pain and the evaluation of new nursing interventions for pain management have been limited by the available measurement technology.

Another common finding is the lack of sufficient conceptual documentation of and explanation for the selection of treatment conditions. This deficiency is manifested in a number of nonproductive studies, despite sound research methodologies. It has been a major concern, particularly for studies including combined cognitive-behavioral strategies. Because pain is complex and involves the application of knowledge from social, behavioral, and biomedical fields, pain research in nursing depends, in part, on how well investigators use existing knowledge from pertinent disciplines.

Type of pain seems to have a significant influence upon pain assessment and management. Therefore, researchers should make greater efforts to identify and control for type of pain in studies. Research within pain categories (e.g., chest, cancer, burn, and postabdominal surgery pain; short-term, long-term, and progressive pain) eventually should bring about a sufficient research base from which practice strategies may be drawn. Other needs in pain research include theory-building on pain conditions and trajectories, variations in patient behavior, cognitive tools, and concepts for pain assessment. It is essential in future research to keep in mind *what* is being measured (e.g., pain threshold, tolerance, or magnitude), as well as *how* it is to be measured. We know that one strategy may affect pain tolerance and not affect threshold, and also that one measure may uncover differences when another does not.

Another variable influencing pain assessment and management was patient age. Apart from several studies indicating that patients' ages affected nurses' inferences of pain, the patient's age was examined in only one study as a principal factor affecting nursing interventions for pain. With increasing knowledge of the developmental stages of adult behavior coupled with an aging population, ongoing study of pain behavior and its relief routinely should include age as a factor.

In this review of research on pain, several consistent findings as to the efficacy of nursing interventions are suggested: (a) the psychosocial components of patients' pain and distress can be altered significantly by nursing interventions and (b) nursing interventions are not effective consistently in reducing patients' pain ratings, with the exception of increased dosage and regular administration of medication. Also, nurses' inferences of patients' pain are not accurate assessments, implying a need for increased work on instrument development as well as for inservice education and training of staff. Conflicting evidence on the effectiveness of interventions may be resolved in part through increased research, although the efficacies of many nursing interventions may depend more upon the particular nurse–patient interaction than upon any inherent differences among the strategies. Also, the study of length of professional nursing experience as a variable affecting nurses' inferences about patients' pain needs to be replicated and extended because it has far-reaching implications for nursing practice.

Another area of pain research that needs considerable development is study of the organizational variables that affect how staff carry out work related to patients' pain. To facilitate such research, more collaborative, multidisciplinary studies are required that focus on complex pain behaviors.

The attention of nurse investigators in the field of pain research in the next two decades (1985–2005) should be directed toward conducting studies in which findings will be cumulative, developing programmatic research endeavors, and obtaining research monies. Through such efforts we will develop the needed empirical evidence for research-based nursing practice in caring for individuals who experience pain.

REFERENCES

Abu-Saad, H. (1984). Assessing children's responses to pain. *Pain, 19*, 163–171.

Anderson, J. L. (1982). Nursing management of the cancer patient in pain: A review of the literature. *Cancer Nursing, 5*, 33–41.

Baer, E., Davitz, L. J., & Lieb, R. (1970). Inferences of physical pain and psychological distress in relation to verbal and nonverbal patient communication. *Nursing Research, 19*, 388–392.

Bagley, C. S., Falinski, E., Garnizo, N., & Hooker, L. (1982). Pain management: A pilot project. *Cancer Nursing, 5*, 191–199.

Beyer, J. E., & Byers, M. L. (1985). Knowledge of pediatric pain: The state of the art. *Children's Health Care, 13*, 150–159.

Beyer, J. E., DeGood, D. E., Ashley, L. C., & Russell, G. A. (1983). Patterns of postoperative analgesic use with adults and children following cardiac surgery. *Pain, 17*, 71–81.

Blitz, B., & Dinnerstein, A. J. (1968). Effects of different types of instruction on pain parameters. *Journal of Abnormal Psychology, 73*, 276–280.

Bochnak, M. A. (1982). The effect of an automatic and deliberative process of nursing activity on the relief of patients' pain: A clinical experiment. In J. A. Horsley (Ed.), *Pain: Deliberative nursing interventions* (pp. 37–60). New York: Grune & Stratton.

Bradford, R. J. (1981). Relationships among marital adjustment, chest pain, and anxiety in myocardial infarction patients. *Issues in Mental Health Nursing, 3*, 381–397.

Bruegel, M. A. (1971). Relationship of preoperative anxiety to perception of postoperative pain. *Nursing Research, 20*, 26–31.

Burckhardt, C. S. (1984). The use of the McGill pain questionnaire in assessing arthritis pain. *Pain, 19*, 305–314.

Carter, B. L. (1967). Comparison of individual pain reactions to injections of distilled water and normal saline. *American Nurses' Association regional clinical conferences* (pp. 219–225). New York: Appleton-Century-Crofts.

Chambers, W. G., & Price, G. G. (1967). Influence of nurse upon effects of analgesics administered. *Nursing Research, 16*, 228–233.

Cohen, M. L. (1980). Postsurgical pain relief: Patients' status and nurses' medication choices. *Pain, 9*, 265–274.

Copp, L. A. (1974). The spectrum of suffering. *American Journal of Nursing, 74*, 491–495.

Copp, L. A. (1985a). Pain coping. In L. A. Copp (Ed.), *Perspectives on pain* (pp. 3–16). Edinburgh: Churchill Livingstone.

Copp, L. A. (1985b). Pain coping model and typology. *Image: The Journal of Nursing Scholarship, 17*, 69–71.

Cunningham, C. L. (1974). The effect of myoelectric feedback on muscle tension and pain experience in patients following discogram and discolysis. *American Nurses' Association clinical sessions* (pp. 279–287). New York: Appleton-Century-Crofts.

Davitz, L. J., & Davitz, J. R. (1975). How nurses view patient suffering. *RN, 38*, 69–74.

Davitz, L. J., & Davitz, J. R. (1981). *Inferences of patients' pain and psychological distress: Studies of nursing behaviors.* New York: Springer Publishing.

Davitz, L. L., Davitz, J. R., & Higuchi, Y. (1977a). Cross-cultural inferences of physical pain and psychological distress—1. *Nursing Times, 73*, 521–523.

Davitz, L. L., Davitz, J. R., & Higuchi, Y. (1977b). Cross-cultural inferences of physical pain and psychological distress—2. *Nursing Times, 73*, 556–558.

Davitz, L. J., & Pendleton, S. H. (1969). Nurses' inferences of suffering. *Nursing Research, 18*, 100–107.

Degner, L. F., Fujii, S., & Levitt, M. (1982). Implementing a program to control chronic pain of malignant disease for patients in an extended care facility. *Cancer Nursing, 5*, 263–268.

Diers, D., Schmidt, R. L., McBride, M. A. B., & Davis, B. L. (1972). The effect of nursing interaction on patients in pain. *Nursing Research, 21*, 419–428.

Dudley, S. R., & Holm, K. (1984). Assessment of the pain experience in relation to selected nurse characteristics. *Pain, 18*, 179–186.

Dunbar, N. (1976). Percutaneous stimulation in the treatment of acute and chronic pain. *Journal of Neurosurgical Nursing, 8*, 105–112.

Eland, J. M. (1985). The role of the nurse in children's pain. In L. A. Copp (Ed.), *Perspectives on pain* (pp. 29–45). Edinburgh: Churchill Livingstone.

Eland, J. M., & Anderson, J. E. (1977). The experience of pain in children. In A. K. Jacox (Ed.), *Pain: A sourcebook for nurses and other health professionals* (pp. 453–473). Boston: Little, Brown.

Engel, G. L. (1959). "Psychogenic" pain and the pain-prone patient. *American Journal of Medicine. 26*, 899–918.

Fagerhaugh, S. Y. (1974). Pain expression and control on a burn care unit. *Nursing Outlook, 22*, 645–650.

Flaherty, G. G., & Fitzpatrick, J. J. (1978). Relaxation technique to increase comfort level of postoperative patients: A preliminary study. *Nursing Research, 27*, 352–355.

Geden, E., Beck, N., Brouder, G., & O'Connell, E. (1983). Identifying procedural components for analogue research of labor pain. *Nursing Research, 32*, 80–83.

Geden, E., Beck, N., Hauge, G., & Pohlman, S. (1984). Self-report and psychophysiological effects of five pain-coping strategies. *Nursing Research, 33*, 260–265.

Grabinski, P. Y. (1983). I.M. injections—Deltoid or gluteal site? *PRN Forum, 2*(3), 1–2.

Graffam, S. R. (1970). Nurse response to the patient in distress—Development of an instrument. *Nursing Research, 19*, 331–335.

Graffam, S. R. (1981). Congruence of nurse–patient expectations regarding nursing in pain. *Nursing Leadership, 4*, 12–15.

Graffam, S. (1984). Report of survey of untoward reactions to relaxation strategies. *PRN Forum, 3*, 3.

Hammond, K. R., Kelly, K., Schneider, R., & Vancini, M. (1966). Clinical inference in nursing. *Nursing Research, 15,* 134–138.

Healy, K. M. (1968). Does preoperative instruction make a difference? *American Journal of Nursing, 68,* 62–67.

Horowitz, B., Fitzpatrick, J. J., & Flaherty, G. (1984). Relaxation techniques for pain relief after open heart surgery. *Dimensions of Critical Care Nursing, 3,* 364–371.

Hunt, J. M., Stollar, T. D., Littlejohns, D. W., Twycross, R. G., & Vere, D. W. (1977). Patients with protracted pain: A survey conducted at the London Hospital. *Journal of Medical Ethics, 3,* 61–73.

Itty, A., Kurian, A., & Cherian, L. (1977). Intramuscular injections. *The Nursing Journal of India, 68,* 251–252.

Jacox, A. K. (1979). Assessing pain. *American Journal of Nursing, 79,* 895–900.

Jacox, A. K., & Stewart, M. (1973). Relation of psychosocial factors and type of pain. In E. M. Jocobi & L. E. Notter (Eds.), *Proceedings of the ninth nursing research conference of the American Nurses' Association* (pp. 13–38). New York: Appleton-Century-Crofts.

Johnson, J. E. (1973). Effects of accurate expectations about sensations on the sensory and distress components of pain. *Journal of Personality and Social Psychology, 27,* 261–275.

Johnson, J. E., & Rice, V. H. (1974). Sensory and distress components of pain: Implications for the study of clinical pain. *Nursing Research, 23,* 203–209.

Johnson, J. E., Rice, V. H., Fuller, S. S., & Endress, M. P. (1981). Sensory information, instruction in a coping strategy, and recovery from surgery. In J. A. Horsley (Ed.), *Preoperative sensory preparation to promote recovery* (pp. 33–60). New York: Grune & Stratton.

Kaempfer, S. H. (1982). Relaxation training reconsidered. *Oncology Nursing Forum, 9,* 15–18.

Kaiko, R. F., Wallenstein, S. L., Rogers, A. G., Grabinski, P. Y., & Houde, R. W. (1982). Narcotics in the elderly. *Medical Clinics of North America, 66,* 1079–1089.

Kim, S. (1980). Pain: Theory, research and nursing practice. *Advances in Nursing Science, 2*(2), 43–59.

Laborde, J. M., & Powers, M. J. (1983). Evaluation of educational interventions for osteoarthritics. *Multiple Linear Regression Viewpoints, 12,* 12–37.

Lenburg, C. B., Burnside, H., & Davitz, L. J. (1970). Inference in physical pain and psychological distress in relation to length of time in the nursing education program. *Nursing Research, 19,* 399–401.

Lenburg, C. B., Glass, H. P., & Davitz, L. J. (1970). Inferences of physical pain and psychological distress in relation to the stage of the patient's illness and occupation of the perceiver. *Nursing Research, 19,* 392–398.

Levin, R. F. (1982). Choice of injection site, locus of control, and the perception of momentary pain. *Image, 14*(1), 26–32.

Locsin, R. G. (1981). The effect of music on the pain of selected postoperative patients. *Journal of Advanced Nursing, 6,* 19–25.

Manderino, M. A., & Bzdek, V. M. (1984). Effects of modeling and information on reactions to pain: A childbirth-preparation analogue. *Nursing Research, 33,* 9–14.

Mason, D. J. (1981). An investigation of the influences of selected factors on nurses' inferences of patient suffering. *International Journal of Nursing Studies, 18,* 251–259.

McBride, M. A. B. (1966). "Pain" and effective nursing practice. *American Nurses' Association clinical sessions* (pp. 75–82). New York: Appleton-Century-Crofts.

McDonald, S. F. (1982). Effect of visible lightwaves on arthritis pain: A controlled study. *International Journal of Biosocial Research, 3*, 49–54.

McGuire, D. (1984). The measurement of clinical pain. *Nursing Research, 33*, 152–156.

Melzack, R. (1975). The McGill pain questionnaire: Major properties and scoring methods. *Pain, 1*, 277–299.

Moore, D. E., & Blacker, H. M. (1983). How effective is TENS for chronic pain? *American Journal of Nursing, 83*, 1175–1177.

Moss, F. T. (1967). The effect of a nursing intervention on pain relief. *American Nurses' Association regional clinical conferences* (pp. 247–254). New York: Appleton-Century-Crofts.

Moss, F. T., & Meyer, B. (1966). The effects of nursing interaction upon pain relief in patients. *Nursing Research, 15*, 303–306.

Mulcahy, R. A., & Janz, N. (1973). Effectiveness of raising pain perception threshold in males and females using a psychoprophylactic childbirth technique during induced pain. *Nursing Research, 22*, 423–427.

Oberst, M. T. (1978). Nurses' inferences of suffering: The effects of nurse-patient similarity and verbalizations of distress. In M. J. Nelson (Ed.), *Clinical perspectives in nursing research* (pp. 38–60). New York: Teachers College Press.

Perez, S. (1984). Reducing injection pain. *American Journal of Nursing, 84*, 645.

Peric-Knowlton, W. (1984). The understanding and management of acute pain in adults: The nursing contribution. *International Journal of Nursing Studies, 21*, 131–143.

Pierce, J., & Ya Deau, R. E. (1980). Methadone for pain relief in disseminated malignant disease. *Oncology Nursing Forum, 7*, 14–17.

Rankin, M. A. (1982). Use of drugs for pain with cancer patients. *Cancer Nursing, 5*, 181–190.

Rankin, M. A., & Snider, B. (1984). Nurses' perceptions of cancer patients' pain. *Cancer Nursing, 7*, 149–155.

Sofaer, B. (1983). Pain relief—the core of nursing practice. *Nursing Times, 79*, 38–42.

Sternbach, R. A. (1975). Psychophysiology of pain. *International Journal of Psychiatry and Medicine, 6*, 63–73.

Stewart, M. L. (1977). Measurement of clinical pain. In A. K. Jacox (Ed.), *Pain: A source book for nurses and other health professionals* (pp. 107–137). Boston: Little, Brown.

Strauss, A., Fagerhaugh, S. Y., & Glaser, B. (1974). Pain: An organizational—work—work—interactional perspective. *Nursing Outlook, 22*, 560–566.

Taylor, A. G., Skelton, J. A., & Butcher, J. (1984). Duration of pain condition and physical pathology as determinants of nurses' assessments of patients in pain. *Nursing Research, 33*, 4–8.

Taylor, A. G., West, B. A., Simon, B., Skelton, J., & Rowlingson, J. C. (1983). How effective is TENS for acute pain? *American Journal of Nursing, 83*, 1171–1174.

Teske, K., Daut, R. L., & Cleeland, C. S. (1983). Relationships between nurses' observations and patients' self-reports of pain. *Pain, 16*, 289–296.

Voshall, B. (1980). The effects of preoperative teaching on postoperative pain. *Topics in Clinical Nursing, 2*, 39–43.

Walike, B. C., & Meyer, B. (1966). Relation between placebo reactivity and selected personality factors: An exploratory study. *Nursing Research, 15*, 119–123.

Watson, D. (1982). Neurotic tendencies among chronic pain patients: An MMPI item analysis. *Pain, 4*, 365–385.

Wells, N. (1982). The effect of relaxation on postoperative muscle tension and pain. *Nursing Research, 31*, 236–238.

Chapter 3

Human Biologic Rhythms

GERALDENE FELTON
COLLEGE OF NURSING
THE UNIVERSITY OF IOWA

CONTENTS

Rhythms consist of recurring events that are called *cycles*. In an effort to explain rhythms as they relate to biologic functions, scientists have developed chronobiology as a discipline over the past 30 years, and now documentation verifies that virtually all measurable physiological, psychological, and environmental variables fluctuate along a measurable time scale (Aschoff, 1965; Bunning, 1967; Conroy & Mills, 1970; Kleitman, 1963) with the most fundamental coordination of these rhythms around the 24-hour cycle of night and day; these 24-hour cycles are called *circadian rhythms*.

Because little, if any, research in biologic rhythms was conducted by nurses prior to 1964, the major data base used in this review was published studies conducted by nurses during the period from 1964 to 1984. Neither unpublished master's theses, doctoral dissertations, nor abstracts are reported. Occasionally research other than nursing research is cited for explanatory purposes. References to the literature were located through computerized retrieval searches using the National Library of Medicine's *Medline*, *Science Citation Index*, and *Excerpta Medica*.

The chapter includes an overview of biologic rhythms, theoretical frameworks for research on rhythmic phenomena, methodological matters in the study of time, and research related to biologic rhythms in health and illness, time perception, and rotating shift work. The chapter concludes with research directions and implications for practice. It should be noted that this chapter is not about biorhythms. According to certain theorists biorhythms consist of three internal cycles — physical, intellectual, and emotional — that govern everyone, beginning on the date of birth, and influencing well-being ever after. There is no experimental evidence to support the existence of biorhythms, and they should not be confused with biologic rhythms.

THEORETICAL FRAMEWORKS FOR
RESEARCH ON RHYTHMIC PHENOMENA

As explained by Shallis (1983), time is experienced in various ways. The passing seconds, days, and years make time seem to flow with its own inertia, carrying everything along with it, including us. Time is perceived also as a succession of moments with a clear distinction between past, present, and future.

Then there are the models of *linear* and *cyclical* time. Separated into its instants or moments, linear time stretches back into the past — marked on a scale of years, decades, centuries — and forward into the future. The view of time as cyclical is based on the various rhythmic characteristics of nature and the repeatability of events: the day, the season, the year. Thus, time becomes the element within which natural events occur. People react to linear, countable time (hours, minutes, and seconds) as well as to the cycle of the day, the week, and the month, experiencing time as the separation of events, the ordering of experience, and the duration between them.

Two ways of describing time as a relation between events are as a quantity and as a quality (Shallis, 1983). The concept of linear time is nicely quantifiable, but it does not allow for a description of the quality of time. The implied difficulties in linking descriptions of quantitative and qualitative time with the meaning of the changing relationship of things and the part time plays in human experience make the efforts of nurse researchers who try to do research on time all the more admirable.

Nurses who have studied biologic rhythm phenomena have used various time and rhythm perspectives to build nursing theory. Several investigators tested the theoretical framework underlying Martha Rogers's life process model of the science and practice of professional nursing. Basic to Rogers's (1970, 1980) model of unitary human development have been conceptualizations of human–environment interaction characterized by rhythms throughout the developmental phases, the movement of holistic man toward increasing complexity and diversity, and changes in patterning and organization evidenced by changes in the associated wave patterns and rhythmic activity identifying the whole. Among the series of studies, four were part of focused research programs in which propositions derived from Rogers's principles were operationalized and the problem pursued further, adding different techniques and methods to measure temporal activity and the perception of time under a variety of conditions.

Newman has attempted to relate the concepts of speed of walking, rate of movement, time experience, time perception, dependency upon movement, and consciousness (Newman, 1972, 1976, 1979, 1982; Newman & Gaudiano, 1984). Floyd (1982, 1983, 1984) has studied biologic rhythms within psychiatric settings to determine the relationships among environmental disruption, sleep–wakefulness patterns, and mental illness; particularly affective illness and the clinical efficacy of various treatment approaches. Fitzpatrick and her students, and colleagues have used a multidimensional approach to study various aspects of rhythmic patterning, motion, temporality, consciousness, and perception in examining crisis experiences, relaxation, and health (Fitzpatrick, 1980, 1982; Fitzpatrick & Donovan, 1978; Fitzpatrick, Donovan, & Johnston, 1980). Fitzpatrick's (Fitzpatrick & Whall, 1983) theoretical framework was derived from classical biologic rhythm theory and Rogers's correlates of human development and functioning (Rogers, 1970, 1980; Floyd, 1983). Pressler (1983) described and analyzed the Fitzpatrick rhythm model for nursing science.

The theoretical framework derived from Felton's continuing work with biologic rhythm phenomena has been sustained by the commonalities perceived among four situations: rapid travel across time zones, the advancement of the clock by one hour in the spring, the modification of the environment during hospitalization or other institutionalization, and the requirement that nurses operate at peak performance no matter what the time of day or night (Felton, 1970, 1973, 1975; Felton & McLaughlin, 1976; Felton & Ward, 1977). There are, of course, recognizable differences in those situations. The modern jet traveler is displaced into a different time zone, whereas the patient or client, the shift worker, and the person living in a culture that moves to daylight saving time change their sleep and activity timetable within the same time zone. However, there is an important common denominator in these situations: the measurable consequences associated with the change of the human organism's sleep and activity pattern away from the point in time to which it has become accustomed. In each instance, rapid shift in time-related referents is the stressor. The result is that internal rhythms shift out of phase with external cues, such as social routine and the sleep–wake cycle, that normally act to synchronize the internal circadian rhythms when the individual is adapted to local clock time.

METHODOLOGICAL MATTERS IN STUDYING BIOLOGIC RHYTHMS

With appropriate numerical methods and displays, the rhythms part of much biologic variability can be analyzed and isolated. The work of those who study human biologic rhythms begins with documentation of periodicities according to a precise methodology that requires frequent and accurate measurement of the particular function under study over a number of interval periods around the clock. In studying the presence of a circadian rhythm in a physical variable or the effects of changes in biologic rhythms, the following methodological prerequisites are imperative. The design requires a small enough interval between measurements for a given subject on any given day and a large enough total number of days of study to observe behavior over several successive cycles. The investigator then obtains sequential data on the variables(s) and determines whether a rhythm characterizes the original data by fitting a cosine curve of the appropriate period to the time series by the method of least squares. The data need not be spaced equally over each cycle of the rhythm under investigation. Based on the results of fitting the theoretical cosine curve to a fixed period, such as 24 hours, the investigator determines the probability value for the fitted curve. If the probability value is 0.05 or less, the fluctuation of the variable being studied is presumed to be cyclic rather than random.

For purposes of analysis, biologic rhythms data are summarized in various ways. One approach is by a time plot of mean values with dispersion indices. Another approach is to use readily available software packages to derive estimates of rhythm parameters in relation to a selected reference point on the time scale, along with their respective confidence intervals (Dixon, 1970). The descriptions provided are as follows: (a) the interval of time it takes to complete a cycle (the *period*); (b) the number of times an event occurs in a period (the *frequency*); (c) the time location of some part of the cycle (the *phase*); (d) the amount or extent of change in the fluctuation in a cycle (the *amplitude*); (e) the peak time of the rhythmic function (the *acrophase*); (f) the displacement of the acrophase along a time scale (*phase-shift*). Such characterization of rhythms allows statistical inference about differences in timing of rhythms caused by the influence of external cues (synchronizer or zeitgeber) or about changes in parameters of one of several frequencies in a single body of rhythm over time (Halberg, 1976; Hoskins, Halberg, Merrifield, & Hillman, 1979; Reinberg & Halberg, 1971; Smolensky et al., 1976; Stephens & Halberg, 1965).

The COSINOR (Halberg, Johnson, Nelson, Runge, & Sothern, 1972) is a multiple regression procedure that determines the cosine curve for a 24-hour period that best fits the observed pattern of values, thus permitting the detection of a rhythm in the analysis of equally or unequally spaced data and the quantitative evaluation of rhythm amplitude and phase. Used primarily because of its statistical tractability, the COSINOR method may not always be applicable and even may lead to wrong interpretation of the data. Harris (1974) has noted that COSINOR analysis is not very sensitive to skewness. Van-Cauter and Huyberechts (1973) conclude that the COSINOR procedure has restricted application as it is intended primarily for the detection of circadian rhythms. These authors noted that the failures of the COSINOR test as a detection method are evidenced by the need to have *a priori* knowledge of the exact frequency of the period of the phenomena under investigation. In other words, the quality of the fitting is damaged if the phenomenon has more than a single known natural frequency. Rather, the authors recommended the periodogram method because it provides a better analysis of the data with regard to detection and estimation. However, the periodogram, which considers each frequency independently, is only applicable if sampling occurs at equal time intervals.

Other investigators have had different experiences related to curve fitting. Horne and Ostberg (1976), particularly interested in individual differences in temperature curves and possible differences in skewness, used the method of least square fitting of algebraic polynomials and employed an algebraic polynomial curve-fitting program. Felton and Ward (1977), using least squares and COSINOR analysis, found that the maximum points of the observed peaks of fitted values for sodium, potassium, creatinine, and osmolality did not cause a smooth curve. One explanation for why the COSINOR method was not good may have been that individuals in the sample were not synchronized in both frequency and phase of their rhythms, and thus difference in individual rhythms obliterated the rhythm as a group phenomenon. Use of a characteristic point in the synchronization schedule, such as a clock hour of commencement of sleep, time of midsleep, or time of termination of sleep (Smolensky et al., 1976) as the phase reference may have compensated better for differences in synchronization among subjects. It also may have compensated for the fact that a specific clock hour may not reflect the same circadian system phase in individuals adhering to subtly dissimilar rest–activity schedules.

BIOLOGIC RHYTHMS IN
HEALTH AND ILLNESS

Usual Patterns of
Circadian Rhythms

The first nursing studies of rhythms were designed during the late 1960s and early 1970s to verify others' findings about circadian rhythms. Stephens and Halberg (1965) used autorhythmometry to study usual phase relationships among mood, time perception, blood pressure, pulse, temperature, and grip strength. Autorhythmometry was the measurement and recording of physiological and psychological variables as a function of time by the self or automatic means and included the inferential statistical estimation of temporal parameters (Halberg et al., 1972). Felton (1970) studied circadian relationships between body temperature and blood pressure in 32 healthy young women before and after the shift to daylight saving time. DeRisi (1968) and Alderson (1974) studied temperatures of hospitalized male patients. DeRisi's work dealt with differences in the occurrence of maximum temperature elevations and hospital twice-daily temperature-taking routines. Alderson studied the effects of increased body temperature on patients' time perception. Tooraen (1972) studied plasma serum cortisol and excretory rhythms of urinary potassium, sodium, and 17-hydroxy corticosteroids in intensive care unit nurses. Earlier, Pride (1968) failed to find a high correlation between self-reported anxiety and urinary potassium. Scientists have revealed that patients reporting high levels of anxiety and discomfort during the earliest stage of admission to intensive care are characterized by increased urinary sodium retention and potassium output, leading to an increasing Na:K ratio value. The latter measure was suggested by Hale, Williams, and Smith (1971) as a more sensitive stress index than either sodium or potassium alone.

Sleep has been one example of a succession of repeated cycles. Using a 10-day recording based on 2-hour observation intervals, Wessler, Rubin, and Sollberger (1976) found a remarkable circadian regularity in their institutionalized subjects 71 to 94 years of age despite opposite expectations. The long recording period allowed for an efficient time series analysis and strengthened the inferences made about the stability of the adjustment process of a regular living regimen. Studying 22 healthy, aged subjects, Hayter (1983) found a significant increase in time in bed, total sleep time when naps were included, number of naps, and amount of naptime after age 75. Hayter's subjects older than 85 years indicated a significant increase in sleep latency, an increase in total sleep time even when naps were excluded, and a change to an earlier bedtime. These findings were confirmed generally by Pacini and Fitzpatrick (1982).

Leddy (1977) was unsuccessful in her attempt to replicate Felton's (1970) work on the effects of modification of sleep time on blood pressure and temperature. The investigator had expected that change of sleep and social routine would clarify whether the environmental routine exerted the dominant influence or whether endogenous timing mechanisms would restore usual internal relationships. Fifty college nursing students were divided into experimental and control groups, with the experimental group assigned a one-hour shift in sleep time. Blood pressure and oral temperature measured at intervals for a period of 10 days showed no evidence of phase shift. However, the lack of support for the hypothesis was due likely to design flaws in the approach to shifting sleep time, mainly in the strategy for requiring that sleep be advanced.

Relatively little has been discovered about circadian variation in children and neonates. Friedeman and Emrich (1978) examined infant sleep–wake patterns and perceptions of 38 mothers aged 21 to 33. Among the instruments were two creative tools developed for use in the subjects' home. The first was designed to obtain data on the mother's preference regarding an ideal wake pattern for her infant. It was used in conjunction with an *Infant Activity Scale* designed to measure the infant's awake time in order to ascertain the discrepancy between ideal and actual sleep–wake patterns each hour during the day. Unfortunately, the psychometric properties of the tools were not discussed. The investigators found that ideal awake time was less than actual awake time and that there was a drop in total hours of reported ideal awake time from delivery to 2 weeks after birth. Discrepancy between actual and ideal awake time decreased over the 3-month study period.

Kuzel (Kuzel et al., 1979; Kuzel, Halberg, & Haus, 1981) reported on selected aspects of investigations of three women from the same family when hormonal and other variables were studied concurrently. The women were in three stages of maturation: the premenarcheal daughter, aged 12; her menstrually cycling mother, aged 35; and the postmenopausal grandmother, aged 60. The subjects were studied by self-measurement several times each day over several weeks on several variables: oral temperature, heart rate, blood pressure, mood, activity, and vigor. Thereafter, each subject was admitted to a clinical research center, placed on bedrest, and had 48-hour sampling of hormones in blood and urine and the recording of temperature, heart rate, and blood pressure. The circadian rhythm characteristics produced by these data were similar to data from matched healthy peer subjects. It was proposed that such reference levels could exemplify how body rhythms can serve as the individual's standard in daily self-monitoring and as baselines in health appraisal for specific therapeutic protocols.

Prinz et al. (1984) studied circadian temperature variations in healthy, aged, adult volunteers and age- and sex-matched patients with Alzheimer's disease. Based on COSINOR analysis measures and unmodified oral temperature data, the findings indicated the presence of normal circadian temperature rhythms in both the healthy, elderly adults and the individuals with mild to moderate Alzheimer's disease. A sex effect showing women higher on temperature than men across time was a finding consistent with sex differences reported for younger populations. The observed circadian variation in temperature was in agreement with other studies demonstrating a normal circadian temperature rhythm in the elderly (Cahn, Folk, & Huston, 1968).

In an area many have wondered about, Nalepka, Jones, and Jones (1983) investigated whether the phase of the moon influences the onset of labor and subsequent infant births. An analysis of data on 3,499 recorded births over 2 years failed to support any such association between influence of full or new moon on incidence of birth.

Disorders of Sleep–Wake Patterns

Many nonnurse scholars have suggested causal relationships in changes in sleep efficiency, mean reduction of sleep before and after surgery, early awakening, delay in sleep onset, increased awakenings, reduction in sleep duration, decreased quality of sleep, and sleep interruptions (Conroy & Mills, 1970; Hollaway, 1977; Kleitman, 1963). Classification of sleep disorders has evolved from analysis of clinical cases as well as from descriptive polygraphic data. Within this comprehensive classification certain major pathophysiological advances were described by Weitzman (1981), including identification of altered sleep stage patterns in major affective illnesses, insomnias related to hypnotic drugs and alcohol, sleep disturbances associated with sleep-induced respiratory impairment, and periodic movements during sleep. Nurse investigators have confirmed that patients experienced a decreased amount of sleep in acute care areas, that environmental factors as well as nursing care interfered with patients' sleep, and that symptoms of postcardiotomy psychosis were evident in patients grossly deprived of sleep (Hagemann, 1981a, 1981b; McFadden & Giblin, 1971; Walker, 1972; Woods, 1972).

Helton, Gordon, and Nunnery (1980) examined the effect of sleep deprivation in 62 critically ill patients during their first 5 days in the intensive care unit (ICU). Measurements included a mental status examination, a sleep interruption check, and calculation of 24-hour potential sleep cycles. The investigators found frequency of mental status changes in the sleep-deprived patients of 33%, a moderate degree of correlation between mental status and interruptions, and confirmation that sleep-deprived subjects were more likely to exhibit symptoms of altered mental states. A like finding of incidence of sleep deprivation in intensive care settings had been reported earlier by Hilton (1976) and supported by Webb and Campbell (1980), whose investigators revealed that decreased quantity and quality of sleep was experienced by more than 70% of ICU patients.

Other investigators have studied sleep during hospitalization and nonhospitalization. In a descriptive study of sleep duration and sleep disruption in hospitalized children 3–8 years old, Hagemann (1981a, 1981b) found that delay in sleep onset produced the greatest loss of sleep. Beardslee (1976) and Pacini and Fitzpatrick (1982), reporting on hospitalized and nonhospitalized elderly, found hospitalized subjects had an average sleep period of from 20% to 25% less than usual, delay in sleep onset, sleep disruption due mostly to caretaking activities, and discomfort early in the sleep period. These findings have potential for adding to the artistry of nursing practice.

Lamb (1982) studied the relationships among newly diagnosed malignancy, anxiety, depression, and sleep, and found that the sleep of the newly diagnosed cancer patient was not significantly different from that of patients who did not have cancer. However, the investigator admitted these results could relate to lack of sensitivity of the sleep assessment tool used.

In a well-conducted study, Parsons and VerBeek (1982) used a self-assessment questionnaire to compare sleep–wake patterns in 75 young male subjects before and after head injury. They found that sleep–wake patterns following head injury differed significantly from those before head injury: Sleep interruptions per night and per week increased, time needed to function at peak efficiency upon awakening increased, number of times per month subjects were unable to return to sleep after early morning awakening increased, quality of sleep decreased, and complaints about sleep increased.

Using a self-assessment questionnaire, Floyd (1984) matched a sample of 35 psychiatric inpatients on gender and psychiatric diagnoses with 35 psychiatric outpatients. The purpose was to explore relationships among subjects' usual time of being asleep and being awake, whether subjects were more active in the morning or in the evening, and subjects' responses to the hospital's rest–activity schedule. She found that hospitalized patients slept less than nonhospitalized patients. However, these differences were not based on subjects' self-reported circadian pattern. The hospitalized subjects experienced phase shifts in their sleep–wake cycles resulting in sleep–wake rhythms that became coupled with the hospital's rest–activity pattern regardless of whether the subjects normally were more active in the morning or the evening. Floyd concluded that this shifting suggested that the hospital routine functions as a strong zeitgeber or synchronizer of sleep and wakefulness.

Circadian Rhythms and
Nursing Practice

Theoretical interest in biologic rhythms has not been followed by much rigorous testing and application of chronobiological methods in nursing practice. One exception was the work of Farr, Keene, Samson, and Michael (1984), which studied circadian changes in temperature among surgical patients; blood pressure; heart rate; and urinary excretion of catecholamine metabolites, 17-ketosteroids, sodium, potassium, and creatinine. Data were examined to determine if a relationship existed between the degree of circadian alteration after surgery and the subject's return to typical circadian profiles. Measurements were made daily at 2-hour intervals on 11 surgery subjects and 10 age- and sex-matched control subjects. The data indicated that certain circadian rhythms of hospitalized subjects were altered and uncoupled from external stimuli.

The Farr et al. (1984) research program has been important because of the expertise the team brings to studying metabolic systems, the careful preliminary work, and Farr's study of computer methods for rhythm analysis under Franz Halberg. The findings from this study suggested that surgery and hospitalization induced changes in the basic circadian rhythmicity of individual subjects, whose rhythms appeared to return toward normal patterns during hospitalization and to a more normal profile during convalescence. However, due to lack of preoperative data and hospital scheduling conflicts in planning of activities such as bathing, ambulation, meals, sleep and wake times, rest periods, medications, and timing of medications, the investigators could not say whether the rhythmic changes were detrimental to patients' recovery. The major importance of this work lay in the potential for better understanding of rhythmic response to stress and trauma. Another aspect of Farr's research was the confirmation that there were considerable differences in the ease and rate at which people's body rhythms accommodated to time shifts.

Moore (1982) used a convenience sample of 13 mildly anxious cancer patients, aged 49 to 68 years, to investigate the influence of time of administration of Cis-platinum on nausea and vomiting. Use of antiemetic drugs and sample characteristics were not controlled. Moreover, the data did not support prior anecdotal reports that patients receiving chemotherapy during evening hours experienced less nausea and vomiting because they "slept off" their symptoms. The study illustrated the influence of individual differences in attempting to make sense of circadian rhythm findings because the results suggested the possibility of predicting individual patterns of nausea and vomiting.

Kuzel's (1973) and her associates' (Halberg et al., 1979; Kuzel, Halberg, & Fozzard, 1981) primary research interest has been the discovery and application of principles of chronobiology. This group has concentrated on the temporal characteristics of cardiovascular functions to determine if a susceptibility phase could be demonstrated in patients with myocardial infarction that was correlated to circadian cycles. Such information would facilitate timed nursing interventions. Data collected for a single 24-hour period on six male subjects admitted to an intensive care unit included hourly measurement of oral temperature and blood pressure and continuous computer monitoring of the electrocardiograph for heart rate and dysrhythmias. Analysis demonstrated statistically significant rhythms with periods of less than 24 hours and the occurrence of cardiac dysrhythmias and premature atrial beats, as well as a circadian rhythmicity in temperature, pulse, respirations, and premature ventricular contractions (PVCs). Studying the time of day for occurrence of PVCs in 10 post myocardial infarction patients Hockenberger and Rubin (1974) were unable to support their hypothesis of PVCs occurring between 1800 hours and 2400 hours. However, this investigation was affected by methodological problems related to accuracy of counting abnormal ventricular contractions, data loss, equipment failure, and lack of a control group.

Studying a random sample of 300 hospital records, O'Donoghue and Rubin (1977) found that postoperative cholecystectomy patients exhibited a time-of-day cycle pattern in the experience of pain. Data collected the first and second postoperative days indicated that the greatest need for pain relief occurred between 2000 hours and midnight. Notwithstanding that such variations may be attibuted to the physiologic effect of circadian variations of plasma cortisol, organizational routines of nursing personnel, and the psychological response of the patient, the findings also may have been influenced by the anticipatory administration of narcotics.

Research has provided evidence that body temperature could be predicted to rise slowly during the day to a high in the mid to late afternoon and then begin to decline. Observation of recorded temperatures has led some investigators to the conclusion that traditional routines of measuring body temperature neither met patients' individual needs nor fit circadian rhythmicity. Moreover, some investigators asserted that besides being a "ritual with no reason," temperature-taking routines used excess human and material resources in nonproductive work. Various suggestions have come from the literature. De-Risi (1968) recommended taking temperatures at 0200 hours, 0600 hours, 1400 hours, 1600 hours and 2200 hours, emphasizing that 1800 hours is the peak time. Schmidt (1972) suggested taking temperatures three times a day in special cases but only once daily otherwise. Sims (1972) concluded that it did no harm to take temperatures at 0700 hours, 1400 hours, and 1900 hours, thus saving nursing effort. In 1965, Stephens and Halberg added to the body of literature that established the stability of body temperature rhythms in normal healthy people. In 1980, Angerami measured axillary temperatures on 255 patients every 2 hours during the day over a period of 8 days. She concluded, as had DeRisi and Schmidt, that for the normal individual taking temperatures once daily at 1900 hours would be sufficient. Problems would arise, of course, if patients were or became hyperthermic. The appropriate criteria to determine when to eliminate temperature measurement have yet to be identified.

Woods and Falk (1974) found relationships among problems of sleep, stress and its concomitant physiological responses, noise levels in the acute care environment, and the number of staff present at patients' bedsides. They also offered suggestions for placement of patients' monitoring and other mechanical equipment, moderation of conversational tones, timing in use of equipment, and design features to deflect noise.

Armstrong-Esther and Hawkins (1982) tried to relate the desynchronization of the circadian system to problems observed in the elderly during hospitalization, such as nocturnal confusion, nocturnal incontinence, and insomnia. Seeking an explanation for the differences between aged and younger persons' response to nature's light-dark cycle, the investigators postulated that the aged person's response was related to pathological changes in the neural pathways between the retina and pineal gland. Believing that the elderly may have lost their responsiveness to light and dark and begun to rely on social synchronizers, the investigators reasoned that the elderly patients had no reliable social cues in a hospital, and, therefore, their body rhythms went out of synchrony. This desynchrony likely would lead to the confusion, incontinence, and sleep disturbance frequently seen in the elderly after admission to a hospital. The findings of the study were equivocal. It may not have been possible to substantiate the original premise about the pineal gland and the retinal neural pathways with the techniques used. Moreover, this investigation was confounded by the individual chronobiological differences prominent in the aged subjects, a finding documented by Weitzman (1981) and Weitzman, Moline, Czeisler, and Zimmerman (1982). Half of the elderly female subjects in the Armstrong-Esther and Hawkins study had altered temperature rhythms; however, not enough details were provided to explore the meaning of that finding.

Circadian Rhythms and
Interpersonal Conflict

Hoskins (1979, 1981; Hoskins et al., 1979) has been the sole nurse investigator identified with the study of circadian patterns of married couples. Hoskins postulated that daily rhythms would predict the relationship of interpersonal conflict to physiological and psychological differences. Her research is based on the theory (Halberg et al., 1972) that rhythms with different frequencies are found at all levels of biologic integration — ecosystem, population, group, individual, organ system, organ, tissue, cell, and subcellular structure. Hoskins labeled her area of research *social chrono-biology*, based on the notion of a cyclical pattern in family relationships. Basic concepts included role perception and role expectation, communication patterns, periodicity in mood, level of activation, physiological rhythms, dissimilarity between partners in morning versus evening orientation, and introversion versus extroversion.

Hoskins utilized the findings of previous investigators (e.g., Halberg et al., 1972) as the theoretical basis for the construction of an Interpersonal Conflict Scale to measure perceived fulfillment of emotional and interaction needs. Alternate forms of equal validity and reliability were developed for repeated measures over time to facilitate identification of conflicting temporal components in relation to body temperature and activation or readiness to respond (Hoskins et al., 1979; Hoskins & Merrifield, 1981). Her (Hoskins, 1979, 1981) investigation of level of activation, body temperature, and interpersonal conflict involved the study of a sample of 16 married couples over a period of 6 weekdays. The theoretical position was detailed carefully and the study was executed carefully. No correlations emerged in the COSINOR analysis between conflict and desynchrony of partners' body temperature rhythms or between conflict and desynchrony of partners' activation rhythms. However, the data revealed that a flattening in the body temperature rhythm occurred when some subjects expressed high levels of perceived conflict.

ORIENTATION TO TIME AND
TIME PERCEPTION

To examine time awareness, temporal patterns, and the experience of time over the adult life span, nurse investigators have mounted elegant studies of human rhythmic patterns of temporality, motion, consciousness, and perception of time. Such a research perspective requires that the investigator consider the human organism as more than an active information processing system in order to refer to purely physiological processes or to describe hypothetical psychological mechanisms. For time to be judged properly, some constant source of stimuli is required that is relatively invariant. Such a source is provided by the stimuli of the physiological and metabolic rhythms of the body as they change in interaction with each other and with outer environments of the body. These stimuli are sufficiently repetitive and similar and occur with sufficient frequency to provide a basis for other time judgments. Moreover, Doob (1971) maintains there must be the capacity to differentiate events as well as to recognize similarities between events.

Requirements for discrimination and memory have led to two major methods for measuring temporal judgment: verbal estimation and production. The concepts of over- and underestimation of time are plagued with confusion, and clock time is the most useful standard for the duration of an interval. Using the verbal estimation method to measure temporal judgment, a subject underestimates a 40-second clock time interval when he says it lasts for 30 seconds; he overestimates the interval when he says it lasts for 50 seconds.

The production method of measuring temporal judgment has been more difficult to understand and interpret. In this approach a subject who is directed to push a button and hold it for 40 seconds underestimates the clock time interval if he holds for 50 seconds; he overestimates the interval by holding for 30 seconds. Newman (1976) has tried to clear up the confusion by indicating that "the data from the production estimate in terms of actual seconds are opposite to the interpretation of the phenomenon occurring, meaning shorter production estimates equal overestimation and longer production estimates equal underestimation (p. 274)."

Nurse investigators have used both production and verbal estimation methods to test event–rate theories. Comparing time estimation of hospitalized patients during febrile and afebrile states, Alderson (1974) and Bell (1965) found that when metabolism was speeded up, as in fever or under great stress, personal (subjective) time was experienced as speeded up, and clock time was overestimated. Collett (1974) used the production method to examine relationships among perceived duration, perceived personal space, and circadian variation in body temperature. However, she was unable to support hypotheses about associations between body temperature and production interval. In an earlier study of perceived duration, Stephens and Halberg (1965) found that the production method yielded a closer estimate for passage of a 120-second elapsed period of clock time than did the verbal estimation method.

Two instruments that were used both by Melillo (1980) and Fitzpatrick (1980) may be useful for other nursing research because the psychometric properties are known: the Time Metaphor Test (Knapp & Garbutt, 1958), which assesses rate of time passage and achievement motive; and the Time Opinion Survey (Kuhlen & Monge, 1968), which elicits attitudes and motives related to time. Data collected with these tools did not provide support for Melillo's hypothesis that a greater number of hours of informal activity was related to a swifter perceived speed of passing time. Methodological refinement may require correlating physiological measures with the two instruments and using a production method of perceived duration.

Newman (1972) used the production method to test whether an imposed alteration in the rate of walking was accompanied by a change in perceived duration. Results failed to support the hypothesis, but Newman interpreted her findings to suggest that individuals with faster gait tempos tended to overestimate an interval of time and those with a slower gait tempo tended to underestimate. In a 1976 study, Newman's hypothesized relationship between preferred rate of walking and perceived duration by production method was not supported, but she found a linear relationship between actual walking rate and perceived duration.

Data from a 1979 study led Newman to believe that an increase in subjective (personal) time indicated an increase in level of consciousness, and that the increase in consciousness was associated with age. Therefore, in her next study (1982) she explored subjective time as a developmental phenomenon of expanding consciousness among 60 to 88-year-old subjects by examining relationships between both age and movement and the perceived duration of a 40-second interval. Subjects produced estimates of 40-second intervals under two conditions: (a) while sitting quietly, and (b) while walking around a prescribed oval track at their preferred rate of walking. Thus, Newman defined consciousness to include the capacity of a system to respond to stimuli as well as judging the passage of clock time. Neither age–time nor movement–time relationships were confirmed. However, in comparing subjective time of younger and older subjects, the investigator postulated an equivocal trend toward the elderly's increasing consciousness with age and an increase in the rate of passage of subjective time. This speedup contradicted the biological assumption that age-related slowing down of metabolism should produce a slowdown in perception of the passage of time. In 1984, Newman and Gaudiano linked depression and time perception in a study of ambulatory elderly women to explain the incongruities between research findings that subjective time increases with age and the fact that metabolism decreases with age. When subjective time was determined by having the subject give an estimate of an interval of 40 seconds, the investigators found little depression but a positive correlation between depression and decreased subjective time, the underestimation of the duration of a 40-second interval. Notwithstanding the demonstrated relationship, the investigators admitted that the study had methodological weaknesses and that procedural improvements were warranted.

The literature provides evidence that temporal behavior varies with age only when changes in the state of the organism vary with age. This means that the correlation existing between age and temporal judgment is rendered imperfect by the obvious fact that changes in behavior are not perfectly correlated with age. The investigator then is caught on the horns of the dilemma of opposing views in the time perception literature. One group claims a linear and positive relationship among the presented stimuli. Hall (1959) states that estimation of the duration of time increases with increased stimulus complexity. An opposing view shows a negative association between the experiential complexity that fills a given interval and assessment of time duration. As a result, a shortened time period is experienced with increased stimulus complexity. An experiential view is that the more actively individuals process environmental stimuli, the more swiftly time seems to pass; whereas, conversely, time seems to pass more slowly when individuals experience given stimuli less actively. The evidence is not overwhelmingly in support of hypotheses that perceptual and motor speed differences associated with increased age can be attributable to a slower perceived rate of the passage of time.

Hogan (1978) maintains that these opposing views can be reconciled by considering time perception as a U-shaped function of both personality and stimulus complexity, rather than as a linear concept. There are many orientations to the study of time, only some of which have been investigated, and perhaps some ways important to nursing theory have not been touched upon. In any event, it may be that a better description of the consequences of time requires better understanding of behavior.

In 1975, Smith first tested the theoretical proposition that humans and environment are in continuing, mutual, and simultaneous interaction and that perception of temporal duration is related to activity, change, and processing of environmental information. With the purpose of exploring the effects of auditory input on bed-confined individuals, Smith had 180 healthy subjects judge the passage of 40-second intervals of time under three different kinds of auditory information during two and a half hours of bed rest. The three kinds of auditory input were intended to be different in patterning, meaning, and intensity. The subjects underestimated the passage of the 40-second intervals; however, in the opinion of the reviewer the main problem arose from the procedures used in the experimental conditions. One of the experimental conditions was not perceived necessarily as an annoying sound, which the investigator had intended. A central problem of auditory perceptions was how the brain interpreted patterns in the receptor organ of the inner ear. The implication was that differences in responses among subjects could have been a function of the experimental condition, but also could have been related to the personality of the subject, as indicated by Blatt and Quinlan (1972).

In two replications, Smith (1979, 1984) studied bed-confined, healthy subjects under different auditory conditions of the ambient environment. In a 1979 study subjects judged duration of a 40-second interval to be greater than 40 seconds of clock time as well as complaining of feeling tired. In a 1984 replication there was no significant difference on the production of a 40-second interval between subjects at rest in a sound-filled environment and those in a quiet, ambient environment. Defining the environment was a problem across the three Smith (1975, 1979, 1984) studies; nonetheless, the findings supported inferences that the temporal potential of an individual could be viewed at the very least as a composite made up of the individual's temporal information and accuracy of temporal judgment. Moreover, the synthesis of ideas, the methods used in planning the experimental conditions, and the instruments devised for Smith's work gave evidence of ingenuity.

In a refinement of Newman's work, Tompkins (1980) tested the relationship between movement and perceived duration, believing that when leg and knee mobility was restricted perceived duration would be likely shortened, and walking would require increased muscular effort. Tompkins used the production method to have subjects judge the passage of 40 seconds of clock time. The data appeared to support the theory that perceived duration was shortened; production judgments were lengthened under conditions of restricted mobility, as compared to perceived duration under the condition of unrestricted mobility and unrestricted preferred walking tempo.

Fitzpatrick and colleagues (Fitzpatrick, 1980, 1982; Fitzpatrick & Donovan, 1978; Fitzpatrick et al., 1980; Fitzpatrick & Whall, 1983) attempted empirically to link perceptions of the passage of time to age, motor activity, and the crisis implied in the diagnosis of terminal illness. Providing an example of careful scholarship, they used instruments with known psychometric properties: the Time Reference Inventory (Roos, 1964); the Time Opinion Survey (Kuhlen & Monge, 1968); the Time Metaphor Test (Knapp & Garbutt, 1958) and the Money Game (Cottle, 1976). The use of Cottle's Circle Test was described, but there was no evidence of its use in Fitzpatrick's published work. What is found are elegant statistical analyses to test relationships among various measures of temporality.

In an attempt to clarify the relationship among time perception, age, and observed body activity, Fitzpatrick and Donovan (1978) studied institutionalized and noninstitutionalized subjects. The institutionalized group was more past-oriented, whereas their noninstitutionalized peers were more present-oriented. Observed differences in body movement in the groups were not considered by the investigators to be significant.

In 1980 Fitzpatrick et al. reported on their analysis to determine if terminally ill cancer patients' perceptions of time varied with the length of time since initial diagnosis of cancer, in comparison to the perceptions of persons not experiencing a health-related crisis. The cancer patients differed temporally from the control subjects in that the cancer group reported a shorter future temporal perspective, more time pressure even though they had more free time, and more curiosity about the time following their death. Few differences were identified on the basis of length of time since diagnosis, except that recently diagnosed patients were more interested in knowing about events that occurred the year preceding their birth. Those diagnosed longer than three years made fewer negative statements about the past.

Other investigators have looked at conceptions of the passage of time and women's temporal experience during labor (Beck, 1983; Butani & Hodnett, 1980; Rich, 1973). The findings confirmed anecdotal reports that women in labor perceived time as moving more slowly.

ROTATING SHIFT WORK

The Department of Labor reports that about one out of four Americans now works a schedule other than the traditional "9-to-5." Estimates are that the percentage is likely to increase in the decade ahead

because the computerization of jobs facilitates round-the-clock operation. Cziesler, Moore, and Coleman (1982) amplify the Department of
Labor statistics by indicating that 26.8% of U.S. workers are required
to rotate work time between days and evenings.

From a physiological point of view, one of the most important
questions is the adaptability of various circadian rhythms to the irreg-
ular and ever-changing pattern of living of the shift worker. Characteristic of these situations is a phase shifting of the working and
sleeping times of between 8 and 12 hours. Consequently, diurnal variations in performance during shift work are linked both to a phase
shifting of performance rhythms and to sleep duration, sleep quality,
and sleep efficiency. Paramount in considering the influence of shift
work on performance, then, is the recognition of the significance of
the reentrainment of physiological and psychological functions to altered sleep–waking schedules. In recent years nurse investigators have
examined this problem mainly in terms of gender, age, drug use
(Floyd, 1983), and physiological functions such as body temperature,
blood pressure, catecholamine excretion, plasma cortisol, urinary
creatinine, potassium, sodium, other cations, and osmolality (Felton,
1973; Hawkins & Armstrong-Esther, 1978; Lanuza & Marotta, 1974;
Tooraen, 1972).

In the Felton study (1973), registered nurses, 21 to 45 years old
and employed in six major hospitals in Hawaii, were required to rotate
work shifts from day (0700 to 1530) to nighttime (2300 to 0730) and
back to daytime. To assure homogeneity, several variables were held
constant: routine of work and recreational activity, age, sex, health
status, diet, time in the local area, and normality of glomerular filtra-
tion rate. For a period of 18 days, interval sampling of body temperature and of urine for potassium, sodium, creatinine, and osmolality
was made every 3 hours from time of awakening until the subject
retired. On night duty subjects had decreased quality and quantity of
sleep, and the time of the temperature and potassium cycle maxima
advanced to a new night duty high, as did that of sodium, creatinine,
and osmolality. These shifts to a later cycle maxima, accompanied by
flattening of the circadian rhythm amplitudes, were statistically significant. All functions showed a one-day lag before advancing to the
night duty level and a comparable lag after night duty, a finding
consistent with other studies. After the subjects rotated from the night
shift back to the day shift, the urinary sodium, creatinine, and osmolality cycles returned to the reference phase relationship with the activ-

ity cycle; temperature and potassium did not return to the reference phase relationship, even after 10 days post-night duty. These findings were supported by the Hawkins and Armstrong-Esther (1978) report that body temperature did not adjust to night work and day sleep even after 7 nights, and Lanuza and Marotta's (1974) conclusions that one week was insufficient time for the nurse to adapt plasma cortisol and cations to a new working schedule, that at physiologic concentrations cortisol did not play a major role in determining cation levels, and that cations affected cortisol levels.

In looking at one individual's circadian pattern, Dwyer, Rubin, and Sollberger (1980) used autorhythmometry to study a diabetic subject who was employed for 3 years, Monday through Friday, on the 2300 to 0730 shift. The investigators examined oral temperature, heart rate, feeling state, hunger, and urinary glucose levels. Admitting to some bothersome problems with the data collection methods, data analysis, and subject adherence to the study protocol, the investigators reported these findings: The subject had weekday inversion of the usual circadian pattern, difficulty in sleeping, decrease in feelings of well-being, and increase in hunger that coincided with decreased body temperature and heart rate and elevated urinary glucose levels. The data provided a basis for altering the time of the subject's daily dosage of insulin.

Comparison of data from different experiments revealed a consistent pattern of associations. Night work and day sleep have been associated with high frequency of sleep complaints, sharply increased difficulties in maintaining sleep, and, as a consequence, experience of sleep as not satisfying. One of the factors not studied by nurses but found to determine people's ability to adjust to shift work may be their degrees of morningness or eveningness (Horne & Ostberg, 1976). Folkard and Monk (1979) were among the investigators who found that the morningness–eveningness scores of subjects correlated with diurnal differences in self-rated alertness, body temperature, and adrenalin secretion.

Because research on shift work has shown that a weekly rotating system is unsatisfactory for the adjustment of circadian rhythms, alternative schedules have been suggested. Permanent shifts, or at least longer spells on the same shift, are suggested to allow a better biological adaptation (Kleitman, 1963; Kleitman & Jackson, 1950; Winget, Hughes, & LaDox, 1978). Because such a system may be unacceptable for social reasons, rotation systems with rapid, rather than slow, alternation have been recommended to reduce both the negative psychosocial and psychological consequences of shift work (Czeisler et al., 1982). Under the rapid alternation rotation, the accumulation of negative effects due to sleep deficit would be minimized; however, an adjustment of circadian rhythm could not be achieved. Slow alternation shift rotation systems have been condemned frequently by chronobiologists as the worst possible form of shift system, sufficient to result in the disruption of circadian rhythms, but insufficient to result in complete adjustment of body rhythms to the inversion of the sleep–wake cycle. Few investigators actually have examined the disruption or adjustment of the circadian rhythms of individual shift workers on the rapid alternation shift rotation system. Perhaps the speed of rotation has been an insufficient criterion for judging the relative merits of different shift rotation systems.

In nursing, variation in shift rotation systems has been tried to minimize burnout, increase job satisfaction, and relieve staffing problems. The 12-hour day has been studied by several investigators. Eaton and Gottselig (1980) determined effects of the 12-hour day on job satisfaction, work environment, nurses' health status, nurses' fatigue and alertness, and quality of patient care. Feichtel-Pascuzzo (1981) studied morale, staffing, communications, continuity, errors, infection, and fatigue. Vik and MacKay (1982) studied effects on patient care. Metcalf (1982) studied whether nurses liked the 12-hour weekend. These investigators found that satisfaction with work, nurses' health, job satisfaction, level of fatigue and alertness, and quality of patient care were not affected unduly by 12-hour shifts, nor were there increased incidents of errors or infection. From these studies the aggregate evidence was overwhelmingly positive that nurses liked 12-hour scheduling for shift rotation. The linking of 12-hour shifts to morale, as these investigators sought to do, encouraged suspicions about external validity. It remained to be seen what role job satisfaction and attitudes toward shift work played in regard to health status, family life, leisure, and social activities.

A little-investigated problem has been night shift paralysis. Never studied by nurses, night shift paralysis may have prevented night workers from performing for several minutes, and, thus, have contributed to problems with safety. This paralysis normally occurred when a nurse performed a sedentary task in the early hours of the morning and then was required to make a gross motor movement. Folkard, Condon, and Herbert (1984) surveyed 434 night nurses to determine the nature of the paralysis, its extent, and its dependence upon age, time of day, and the number of consecutive nights the nurse had worked. Twelve percent of the respondents claimed to have suffered from a totally incapacitating paralysis at least once or twice, occurring around 0400 hours, when the night workers' rated alertness, body temperature, and many psychological and physiological functions were at a low ebb. The incidence of the paralysis was a function of the number of consecutive night shifts the nurse worked. It tended to increase over consecutive night shifts and was confined largely to nurses below the age of 30.

MENTAL EFFICIENCY AND
HUMAN PERFORMANCE

Circadian rhythms in performance have been documented for a wide range of tasks studied under laboratory conditions; they also occurred in measures of efficiency obtained in real life situations. Hildebrandt and Stratmann (1979) and Rutenfranz and Colquhoun (1979) believed that differences between performance levels at different times of day were related to the daily cycle of sleep need because the largest negative variations in performance normally were observed when sleep need was greatest. Evidence from research on morningness and eveningness revealed that there were times in the 24-hour period in which performance was relatively high. When these times were interrupted by periods of increasing sleep need, performance gradually diminished, and sleep and performance were seen as antagonistic phenomena. The literature contained evidence that under experimental conditions with a normal sleep–wake cycle, performance reached its maximum during the afternoon and its minimum in the early morning hours. Different types of stressors, such as changes in sleep–wake cycle, multiple time zone transition, and sleep deprivation, have induced changes in the circadian rhythms (Hockey & Colquhoun, 1972).

Little research has been done on nursing work performance, replete as it is with multiple stressors. These stressors derive from problem-solving and decision-making tasks; perceptional tasks, such as signal detection, monitoring, and vigilance; processing and information-storage tasks; interpersonal coordination and cooperation tasks; and motor skill tasks. The motor skill tasks alone may involve psychic and physical stress that is excessive in intensity, kind, and duration. These stressors may give rise to a state of fatigue. As in aerospace medicine research (Hale et al., 1971; Rotondo, 1978), in nursing work it is possible to identify a number of different components: (a) a physical component, the result of motor, perceptual, or neuromuscular work; (b) a psychic component, the result of mental work and prolonged psychic tension; and (c) an emotional component, the result of exposure to repeated and intense emotions inevitably connected with nurse performance. There is obvious need to analyze the nature of the various stressing and fatiguing factors that act on the body and psyche of nurses and the functional changes that fatigue can produce. However, studies of influences on performance of the many different and complex tasks carried out by nurses are practically nonexistent, and investigations in this area are needed badly.

Body temperature has been a great predictor of performance efficiency (Colquhoun, Blake, & Edwards, 1968a, 1968b; Kleitman, 1963), implying that body temperature is an indicant of the underlying state of arousal of the organism. One question for study concerns what happens to performance and, concurrently, to job efficiency when phases of the body temperature rhythm and other physiological rhythms shift as a result of work shift rotation.

To test the underlying relationship between body temperature and performance, Hawkins and Armstrong-Esther (1978) measured short-term memory tasks and temperatures on 11 nurse subjects. Error scores indicated that the time of lowest temperature correlated with the time of maximum error scores for the first 4 nights of the 7-day test period. Unfortunately, questions can be raised about the general method of analysis. The investigators computed average unadjusted scores for each time interval, thus obliterating the considerable amount of variation between subjects, intra-individual differences, the variability in performance efficiency, and the relationship of this variability to concurrent changes in body temperature. No data were presented on the characteristics of curve forms, amplitudes, time of crest, habitual phase differences in activity patterns, or other important parameters.

SUMMARY, RESEARCH DIRECTIONS, AND IMPLICATIONS FOR PRACTICE

Several features of biological rhythmicity and the circadian system especially have potential importance for nursing research and nursing practice. A high degree of temporal order characterizes the healthy organism. There is adequate documentation of circadian physiological and psychological patterns. There is documentation of phase-dependent differences both in the effectiveness of drugs and in human responses to other stimuli. Research has shown that a discrepancy between the activity schedule of the individual and the environmental schedule can result in psychological and physiological distress and in less efficient performance. The relevance of biologic rhythm research for nursing practice is directed toward the long-term goal of examining nursing measures in light of circadian variations in human physiological and psychological rhythms, changes in timing of rhythm characteristics, ways nurses can control forces that cause desynchronization, and timely intervention to help people to avoid circadian disorganization or to return to typical rhythmic patterns. For instance, sleep research provides much information for testing nursing management of problems of sleep induction and maintenance, altered sleep stages, and insomnia.

Circadian variations in performance have occurred in a wide range of tasks. Although such variations can be influenced by factors such as fatigue, nutrition, and individual differences, available evidence suggests that the observed fluctuations reflect an underlying 24-hour rhythm analogous to those shown by physiological processes that may be closely connected with the cycle of sleep need. Parenthetically, performance rhythms in work settings often are masked by motivational and situational factors. Measurements of performance taken during night hours are confounded by sleep deprivation or sleep interruption. In any case, the study of such situations is of considerable practical interest in nursing and clearly has direct application to the problem of night shift work.

Research has led to various recommendations directed at chronohygiene (Halberg, 1976). Winget et al. (1978) recommended that employers change workers' shifts infrequently, usually no more than once a month, to assure optimum performance and lessen the chance of worker error. Czeisler et al. (1982) recommended that changes in work shift be done in a way that delays the body's natural rhythms rather than advancing them. In other words, a person on the 1500 to 2300 hour shift should be switched to the 2300 to 0700 hour shift on the next rotation instead of the 0700 to 1500 hour shift.

Although night and shift work represented classical problems of chronohygiene, the pathological consequences and the ways to ameliorate the effects of shift work neither have been characterized sufficiently nor tested sufficiently. Blatt and Quinlan (1972) believed that individual differences in the ease and rate at which different people adapted to changes in temporal referents may have been related to important aspects of personality, and have represented stable individual patterns for interacting with the environment. The aspects the investigators identified that caused interindividual variation in the ease and rate at which people's body rhythms accommodated to time shifts were: (a) temporal organization, meaning the rigidity or flexibility of a person's temporal structure for punctuality or procrastination; (b) flexibility of sleep patterns and circumstances necessary for sleep; (c) time of maximum efficiency, meaning whether the individual was a morning person or evening person; and (d) degree to which the individual was responsive to internal physical states or environmental factors, meaning whether the person was field dependent or field independent.

In any case, knowledge of changes in circadian and other biologic systems gives evidence of being a useful nursing research and diagnostic tool. Moreover, research in biologic rhythm phenomena offers the opportunity to bring research in clinical nursing practice more rapidly to a high level of sophistication.

REFERENCES

Alderson, M. (1974). Effect of increased body temperature on the perception of time. *Nursing Research, 23*, 42–49.

Angerami, E. L. S. (1980). Epidemiological study of a body temperature in patients in a teaching hospital. *International Journal of Nursing Studies, 17*, 91–99.

Armstrong-Esther, C. A., & Hawkins, L. H. (1982). Day for night, circadian rhythms in the elderly. *Nursing Times, 78*, 1263–1265.

Aschoff, J. (1965). Circadian rhythms in man. *Science, 148*, 1427–1432.

Beardslee, C. (1976). The sleep-wakefulness pattern of young hospitalized children during nap time. *Maternal-Child Nursing Journal, 5*, 15-24.

Beck, C. T. (1983). Parturients' temporal experiences during the phases of labor. *Western Journal of Nursing Research, 5*, 283-294.

Bell, C. R. (1965). Time estimation and increases in body temperature. *Journal of Experimental Psychology, 70*, 323-324.

Blatt, S. J., & Quinlan, D. M. (1972). The psychological effects of rapid shifts in temporal referents. In J. T. Fraser, F. C. Haber, & G. H. Muller (Eds.), *The study of time* (pp. 506-522). New York: Springer-Verlag.

Bunning, E. (1967). *The physiological clock.* New York: Springer-Verlag.

Butani, P., & Hodnett, E. (1980). Mothers' perceptions of their labor experiences. *Maternal-Child Nursing Journal, 9*, 73-82.

Cahn, H. A., Folk, G. E., & Huston, P. E. (1968). Age comparison of human day-night physiological differences. *Aerospace Medicine, 10*, 608-610.

Collett, B. A. (1974) Variation in body temperature, perceived duration and perceived personal space. *International Journal of Nursing Studies, 11*, 47-60.

Colquhoun, W. P., Blake, M. J. F., & Edwards, R. S. (1968a). Experimental studies of shift work I: A comparison of "rotating" and "stabilized" 4-hour shift systems. *Ergonomics, 11*, 437-453.

Colquhoun, W. P., Blake, M. J. F., & Edwards, R. S. (1968b). Experimental studies of shift work II: Stabilized 8-hour shift systems. *Ergonomics, 11*, 527-546.

Conroy, R. T. W. L., & Mills, J. W. (1970). *Human circadian rhythms.* London: Churchill.

Cottle, T. J. (1976). *Perceiving time.* New York: Wiley.

Czeisler, C. A., Moore, E. M. C., & Coleman, R. M. (1982). Rotating shift work schedules that disrupt sleep are improved by applying circadian principles. *Science, 217*, 460-463.

DeRisi, L. (1968). Body temperature measurements in relation to circadian rhythmicity in hospitalized male patients. *American Nurses' Association Clinical Sessions* (pp. 251-258). New York: American Nurses Association.

Dixon, W. (1970). *BMD Biomedical Computer Programs.* (University of California Publication in Automatic Computation, #2). Berkeley: University of California Press.

Doob, L. W. (1971). *Patterning of time.* New Haven, CT: Yale University Press.

Dwyer, J., Rubin, M., & Sollberger, A. (1980). Clinical autorhythmometry for a diabetic. *Journal of Interdisciplinary Cycle Research, 11*, 179-193.

Eaton, P., & Gottselig, S. (1980). Effects of longer hours, shorter week for intensive care nurses. *Dimensions of Health Services, 57*(8), 25-27.

Farr, L., Keene, A., Samson, D., & Michael, A. (1984). Alterations in circadian excretion of urinary variables and physiological indicators of stress following surgery. *Nursing Research, 33*, 140-146.

Feichtel-Pascuzzo, S. (1981). The 12-hour day. *Nursing Life, 1*, 56-59.

Felton, G. (1970). Effect of time cycle changes on blood pressure and temperature in young women. *Nursing Research, 19*, 48-58.

Felton, G. (1973). Rhythmic correlates of shift work. In M. V. Batey (Ed.), *Communicating nursing research: Vol. 6, The many sources of nursing knowledge* (pp. 73-89). Boulder, CO: Western Interstate Commission on Higher Education.

Felton, G. (1975). Body rhythm effects of rotating work shifts. *Journal of Nursing Administration, 5*(3), 16-19.

Felton, G., & McLaughlin, F. (1976). The collaborative process in generating a nursing research study. *Nursing Research, 25*, 115-120.

Felton, G., & Ward, J., Jr. (1977). Regression models in the study of circadian rhythms in nursing research. *The International Journal of Nursing Studies, 14*, 151-161.

Fitzpatrick, J. J. (1980). Patients' perceptions of time: Current research. *International Nursing Review, 27*, 148-153.

Fitzpatrick, J. J. (1982). The crisis perspective: Relationship to nursing. In J. J. Fitzpatrick, A. L. Whall, R. L. Johnston, & J. A. Floyd (Eds.), *Nursing models and their psychiatric-mental health applications* (pp. 19-35). Bowie, MD: Brady.

Fitzpatrick, J. J., & Donovan, M. J. (1978). Temporal experience and motor behavior among the aging. *Research in Nursing and Health, 1*, 60-68.

Fitzpatrick, J. J., Donovan, M. J., & Johnston, R. L. (1980). Experience of time during the crisis of cancer. *Cancer Nursing, 3*, 191-194.

Fitzpatrick, J. J., & Whall, A. L. (1983). Overview of nursing models and nursing theories. In J. J. Fitzpatrick & A. L. Whall (Eds.), *Conceptual models of nursing* (pp. 1-10). Bowie, MD: Brady.

Floyd, J. A. (1982). Rhythm theory: Relationship to nursing conceptual models. In J. J. Fitzpatrick, A. L. Whall, R. L. Johnston, & J. A. Floyd (Eds.), *Nursing models and their psychiatric-mental health applications* (pp. 95-116). Bowie, MD: Brady.

Floyd, J. A. (1983). Research using Rogers' conceptual system: Development of a testable theorem. *Advances in Nursing Science, 5*, 37-48.

Floyd, J. A. (1984). Interaction between personal sleep-wake rhythms and psychiatric hospital rest-activity schedule. *Nursing Research, 33*, 255-59.

Folkard, S., Condon, R., & Herbert, M. (1984). Night shift paralysis. *Experientia, 40*, 510-512.

Folkard, S., & Monk, T. (1979). Towards a predictive test of adjustment to shift work. *Ergonomics, 22*, 79-91.

Friedeman, M. L., & Emrich, K. A. (1978). Emergence of infant sleep-wake patterns in the first three months after birth. *International Journal of Nursing Studies, 15*, 5-16.

Hagemann, V. (1981a). Night sleep of children in a hospital. Part I: Sleep duration. *Maternal-Child Nursing Journal, 10*, 1-13.

Hagemann, V. (1981b). Night sleep of children in a hospital. Part II: Sleep disruption. *Maternal-Child Nursing Journal, 10*, 127-142.

Halberg, F. (1976). Chronobiology in 1975. *Chronobiologia, 3*, 1-11.

Halberg, F., Haus, E., Kuzel, M., Lakatua, D., Kawasaki, T., Ueno, M., Uezeno, K., Omae, T., Knapp, E., & Gunther, R. (1979). Cost-effective chronobiological monitoring. In A. Albertini, M. DePrade, & B. A. Peskar (Eds.), *Radioimmunoassay of drugs and hormones in cardiovascular medicine* (pp. 107-210). Amsterdam, The Netherlands: Elsevier North Holland Biomedical Press.

Halberg, F., Johnson, E. A., Nelson, W., Runge, W., & Sothern, R. (1972). Autorhythmometry—Procedures for physiologic self-measurements and their analysis. *The Physiology Teacher, 1*, 1-11.

Hale, H. B., Williams, E. W., & Smith, B. N. (1971). Excretion patterns of air traffic controllers. *Aerospace Medicine, 42*, 127.

Hall, E. T. (1959). *The Silent Language.* Greenwich, CT: Fawcett.

Harris, E. K. (1974). Comments on statistical methods for analysing biological rhythms. In L. E. Scheving, D. F. Halberg, & J. E. Pauley (Eds.), *Chronobiology* (pp. 757–760). Tokyo: Igaku Shoin.

Hawkins, L. H., & Armstrong-Esther, C. A. (1978). Circadian rhythms and night shift working in nurses. *Nursing Times, 74*, 49–52.

Hayter, J. (1983). Sleep behaviors of older persons. *Nursing Research, 32*, 242–246.

Helton, M., Gordon, S., & Nunnery, S. (1980). The correlation between sleep deprivation and the intensive care unit syndrome. *Heart and Lung, 9*, 464–468.

Hildebrandt, G., & Stratmann, I. (1979). Circadian system response to night work in relation to the individual circadian phase position. *International Archives of Occupational and Environment Health, 43*, 73–83.

Hilton, B. A. (1976). Quantity and quality of patients' sleep and sleep-disturbing factors in a respiratory intensive care unit. *Journal of Advanced Nursing, 1*, 453–468.

Hockenberger, J. M., & Rubin, M. B. (1974). Cyclic occurrence of premature ventricular contractions in acute myocardial infarction patients: A pilot study. *Nursing Research, 23*, 489–491.

Hockey, G. R., & Colquhoun, W. P. (1972). Diurnal variations in human performance: A review. In W. P. Colquhoun (Ed.), *Aspects of human efficiency — Diurnal rhythm and loss of sleep* (pp. 1–23). London: English Universities Press.

Hogan, W. H. (1978). A theoretical reconciliation of competing views of time perception. *American Journal of Psychology, 91*, 417–428.

Hollaway, F. A. (1977). Overview of research in bio-behavioral rhythms. *Biological Psychological Bulletin, 5*, 39–41.

Horne, J. A., & Ostberg, S. (1976). A self-assessment questionnaire to determine morningness–eveningness in human circadian rhythms. *International Journal of Chronobiology, 4*, 97–110.

Hoskins, C. N. (1979). Level of activation, body temperature and interpersonal conflict in family relationships. *Nursing Research, 28*, 154–160.

Hoskins, C. N. (1981). Psychometrics in nursing research: Construction of an interpersonal conflict scale. *Research in Nursing and Health, 4*, 243–249.

Hoskins, C. N., Halberg, F., Merrifield, P. R., & Hillman, D. C. (1979). Social chronobiology: Circadian activation rhythms of married couples. *Psychological Reports, 45*, 607–614.

Hoskins, C. N., & Merrifield, P. (1981). *Interpersonal conflict scale.* Saluda, NC: Family Life.

Kleitman, N. (1963). *Sleep and wakefulness.* Chicago: University of Chicago Press.

Kleitman, N., & Jackson, D. P. (1950). Body temperature and performance under different routines. *Journal of Applied Physiology, 3*, 309–328.

Knapp, R., & Garbutt, J. (1958). Time imagery and the achievement motive. *Journal of Personality, 26*, 426–434.

Kuhlen, R., & Monge, R. (1968). Correlates of estimated rate of time passage in the adult years. *Journal of Gerontology, 23*, 427–433.

Kuzel, M. (1973). Circadian and ultradian rhythms identified in temperature, blood pressure, heart rate, dysrhythmias, and susceptibility cycles following acute myocardiac infarction. *Circulation, 7, 8,* (Suppl. 4), 235.

Kuzel, M., Frantz, I., Lakatua, D., Kuba, K., Halberg, F., & Haus, E. (1979). Individualized circadian lipid and hormonal rhythmometry of grandmother and granddaughter. *Proceedings of the Minnesota Academy of Science* (p. 15). St. Paul, MN: Minnesota Academy of Science.

Kuzel, M., Halberg, F., & Fozzard, H. (1981). Chronobiological cardiovascular monitoring after myocardial infarction. In C. A. Walker, K. F. A. Soliman, & C. M. Winget, (Eds.), *Chronopharmacology and Chronotherapeutics* (pp. 145-158). Tallahassee: Florida A & M University.

Kuzel, M., Halberg, F., & Haus, E. (1981). Comparison of circadian rhythms in plasma hormones in a daughter, her mother, and grandmother. *International Journal of Chronobiology, 7,* 270.

Lamb, M. A. (1982). The sleeping patterns of patients with malignant and non-malignant diseases. *Cancer Nursing, 5,* 389-396.

Lanuza, D. M., & Marotta, S. F. (1974). Circadian and basal interrelationships of plasma cortisol and cations in women. *Aerospace Medicine, 45,* 864-686.

Leddy, S. (1977). Sleep and phase shifting of biological rhythms. *International Journal of Nursing Studies, 14,* 137-150.

McFadden, E. H., & Giblin, E. C. (1971). Sleep deprivation in patients having open heart surgery. *Nursing Research, 20,* 249-254.

Melillo, K. D. (1980). Informal activity involvement and the perceived rate of time passage for an older institutionalized population. *Journal of Gerontological Nursing, 6,* 392-397.

Metcalf, L. (1982). The 12-hour weekend plan — Does the nursing staff really like it? *Journal of Nursing Administration, 12*(10), 16-19.

Moore, J. M. (1982). The influence of the time of administration on Cis-platinum induced nausea and vomiting. *Oncology Nursing Forum, 9,* 26-32.

Nalepka, C. D., Jones, S. L., & Jones, P. K. (1983). Time variations, births, and lunar association. *Issues in Comprehensive Pediatric Nursing, 6,* 81-89.

Newman, M. A. (1972). Time estimation in relation to gait tempo. *Perceptual Motor Skills, 34,* 359-366.

Newman, M. A. (1976). Movement tempo and the experience of time. *Nursing Research, 25,* 273-279.

Newman, M. A. (1979). *Theory development in nursing.* Philadelphia: F. A. Davis.

Newman, M. A. (1982). Time as an index of expanding consciousness with age. *Nursing Research, 31,* 290-293.

Newman, M. A., & Gaudiano, J. K. (1984). Depression as an explanation for decreased subjective time in the elderly. *Nursing Research, 33,* 137-139.

O'Donoghue, C., & Rubin, M. (1977). *Proceedings, XII International Conference, International Society for Chronobiology* (pp. 365-368). Milan, Italy: The Publishing House.

Pacini, C. M., & Fitzpatrick, J. J. (1982). Sleep patterns of hospitalized and nonhospitalized aged individuals. *Journal of Gerontological Nursing, 8,* 327-332.

Parsons, L. C., & Ver Beek, D. (1982). Sleep-awake patterns following cerebral concussion. *Nursing Research, 31,* 260-264.

Pressler J. (1983). Fitzpatrick's rhythm model: Analysis for nursing science. In J. Fitzpatrick & A. Whall (Eds.). *Conceptual models of nursing* (pp. 303–322). Bowie, MD: Brady.

Pride, L. F. (1968). An adrenal stress index as a criterion measure for nursing. *Nursing Research, 17*, 292.

Prinz, P. N., Christie, C., Smallwood, R., Vitaliano, P., Bokan, J., Vitiello, M. V., & Martin, D. (1984). Circadian temperature variation in healthy aged and in Alzheimer's disease. *Journal of Gerontology, 39*, 30–35.

Reinberg, A., & Halberg, F. (1971). Circadian chronopharmacology. *American Review of Pharmacology, 2*, 455–492.

Rich, O. J. (1973). Temporal and spatial experience as reflected in the verbalizations of multiparous women during labor. *Maternal–Child Nursing Journal, 2*, 239–325.

Rogers, M. E. (1970). *An introduction to the theoretical basis of nursing.* Philadelphia: F. A. Davis.

Rogers, M. E. (1980). Nursing: A science of unitary man. In J. P. Riehl & C. Roy (Eds.), *Conceptual models for nursing practice* (2nd ed.) (pp. 329–337). New York: Appleton-Century-Crofts.

Roos, P. (1964). *Time reference inventory.* Austin, TX: Austin State School.

Rotondo, G. (1978). Wordload and operational fatigue in helicopter pilots. *Aviation, Space and Environmental Medicine, 6*, 430–436.

Rutenfranz, J., & Colquhoun, W. P. (1979). Circadian rhythms in human performance. *Scandinavian Journal of Work Environments and Health, 5*, 167–177.

Schmidt, A. J. (1972). TPRs: An old habit or a significant routine? *Hospitals, 46*, 57–60.

Shallis, M. (1983). *On Time.* New York: Shocker.

Sims, R. S. (1972). Temperature recording in a teaching hospital. *Lamp, 29*, 36–38.

Smith, M. J. (1975). Changes in judgment of duration with different patterns of auditory information for individuals confined to bed. *Nursing Research, 24*, 93–98.

Smith, M. J. (1979). Duration experience for bed-confined subjects: A replication and refinement. *Nursing Research, 28*, 139–144.

Smith, M. J. (1984). Temporal experience and bed rest: Replication and refinement. *Nursing Research, 33*, 298–302.

Smolensky, M. H., Tatar, S. E., Bergman, S. A., Losman, J. G., Barnard, C. N., Dacso, C. C., & Kraft, I. A. (1976). Circadian rhythmic aspects of human cardiovascular function: A review by chronobiologic statistical methods. *Chronobiologia, 3*, 337–371.

Stephens, G., & Halberg, F. (1965). Human time estimation: A study with special reference to 24-hour synchronized circadian rhythms. *Nursing Research, 14*, 310–317.

Tompkins, E. S. (1980). Effect of restricted mobility and dominance on perceived duration. *Nursing Research, 29*, 333–339.

Tooraen, L. A. (1972). Physiological effects of shift and rotation of intensive care nurses. *Nursing Research, 21*, 398–405.

VanCauter, E., & Huyberechts, S. (1973). Problems in the statistical analysis of biological time series: The cosinor test and the periodogram. *Journal of Interdisciplinary Cycle Research, 4*, 41–57.

Vik, G., & MacKay, C. (1982). How does the 12-hour shift affect patient care? *Journal of Nursing Administration, 12*(1), 11–14.

Walker, B. B. (1972). Postsurgery heart patient: Amount of uninterrupted time for sleep and rest during the first, second, and third postoperative days in a teaching hospital. *Nursing Research, 21*, 164–169.

Webb, W. B., & Campbell, S. S. (1980). Awakenings and return to sleep in an older population. *Sleep, 3*, 41–46.

Weitzman, E. D. (1981). Sleep and its disorders. *Annual Review of Neuroscience, 4*, 381–417.

Weitzman, E. D., Moline, M. L., Czeisler, C. A., & Zimmerman, J. C. (1982). Chronobiology of aging: Temperature, sleep–wake rhythms and entrainment. *Neurobiology of Aging, 3*, 299–309.

Wessler, R., Rubin, M., & Sollberger, A. (1976). Circadian rhythm of activity and sleep-wakefulness in elderly institutionalized persons. *Journal of Interdisciplinary Cycle Research, 7*, 333–348.

Winget, C. M., Hughes, L., & LaDox, J. (1978). Physiological effects of rotational work shifting: A review. *Journal of Occupational Medicine, 20*, 204–210.

Woods, N. F. (1972). Patterns of sleep in postcardiotomy patients. *Nursing Research, 21*, 347–353.

Woods, N. F., & Falk, S. A. (1974). Noise stimuli in the acute care area. *Nursing Research, 23*, 144–150.

Chapter 4

Physiologic Responses in Health and Illness: An Overview

MI JA KIM

COLLEGE OF NURSING
UNIVERSITY OF ILLINOIS AT CHICAGO

CONTENTS

Physiologic responses are implicit components of human responses to actual and potential health problems that nurses diagnose and treat (American Nurses' Association, 1980, p. 9). For this chapter, physiologic responses are defined as mechanisms of physical functioning in healthy conditions and functional responses in illness. The work of nurse physiologists and nurse scientists is reviewed in selected areas: cardiovascular, gastrointestinal, respiratory, and neurologic and neuroendocrine systems. Clinical studies of neonatal nursing also are included to represent research on younger populations. The approach used in this chapter is different from that of Lindsey (1982, 1983,

Tables summarizing the distribution of articles by journal and by the review categories are available from the author. Requests should be sent to Mi Ja Kim, Interim Associate Dean for Research, The University of Illinois College of Nursing, Box 6998, Chicago, IL 60680.

79

1984), whose review of research on physiologic phenomena is organized around categories related to the individual, the individual's environment, and nursing therapeutics.

A multistaged process was used to identify potential studies for the review. Lists of nurse physiologists provided by Barbara Hansen and Margaret Heitkemper and American Nurses' Association (1984) rosters were used to identify potential authors and, eventually, physiologically oriented studies in the medical–surgical nursing area. Through this data base and a *MEDLINE* search based on the authors' names, 279 research-related articles were identified. Of those publications, 210 were published in 92 different basic science journals, and 69 were published in 11 different nursing journals. As expected, the majority of studies about the mechanisms of physical functioning came from basic science or nonnursing clinical research journals, whereas most clinical studies came from nursing research journals. One hundred eighty-five articles were excluded because: (a) they were published in other types of journals than physiology, clinical investigation, or nursing; (b) they had limited relevance for nursing; (c) they did not fit into the categories developed for this review; or (d) they were not reports of original investigations. The excluded articles were literature reviews, case studies, abstracts, surveys, or chart reviews. Ninety-four articles were retained for review in the designated categories: cardiovascular, gastrointestinal, respiratory, and neurologic and neuroendocrine systems; and neonatal nursing.

CARDIOVASCULAR SYSTEM

Although nurses studied a wide range of physiologic phenomena, a preponderance of their research efforts were focused on the cardiovascular system. From this broad population of studies, 33 were selected according to the aforementioned criteria.

In 25 studies, researchers dealt with mechanisms of function of the cardiovascular system, including cardiac and skeletal muscles; the remaining eight were studies of the cardiovascular response to a variety of interventions, such as exercise and relaxation. Cowan and her colleagues (Cowan, Reichenbach, Bruce, & Fisher, 1982) demonstrated that the changes in the QRS wave form of an electrocardiogram

(EKG), specifically the integral of the vector spatial magnitudes during the initial abnormal depolarization period, could predict infarct size. The study was done postmortem with 25 patients with myocardial infarction (MI) and 10 controls. In another project, Cowan, Bruce, and Reichenbach (1984) studied 15 patients at necropsy with single inferobasal MIs and 10 patients without heart disease. They showed that the size of transmural infarcts located in the basal inferior, middle inferior, lateral, and inferoseptal left ventricular walls could be estimated by the integral of the spatial magnitudes of sequential vectors during late activation. Findings from these studies indicated that the late activation of the QRS complex may be a better estimate of the left ventricular inferobasal MI size than the abnormalities commonly noted during early activation, that is, during the Q wave. For nurses in cardiac care units who analyze the EKG as a part of their routine assessments of a patient's condition, careful monitoring of the late activation of the QRS complex in relation to spatial vector cardiography may help to identify an extending myocardial infarct and to take the necessary action to minimize the impending complication.

The relationship between the occurrence of premature ventricular contractions (PVCs) and the time of day in which they occur was examined over a 4-day period in 10 patients with an uncomplicated anterior transmural acute myocardial infarct (Hockenberger & Rubin, 1974). Fewer PVCs occurred between 12:00 midnight and 6:00 a.m. Fewer PVCs were noted on the fourth day than on other days. More PVCs occurred between 12:00 noon and 6:00 p.m. Investigators stated that the prophylactic administration of antiarrhythmic drugs may be indicated during the peak time of PVC occurrence. However, other confounding variables, such as age, severity of MI, number of previous MIs, and drugs other than xylocaine hydrochloride and their dosages need to be considered in making a firm recommendation. One needs to be even more cautious in interpreting the results of this study because the sample was small and included only patients who were on xylocaine hydrochloride.

Donaldson and her associates focused on the area of cardiac and skeletal muscle function. It must be noted that Donaldson's research program is described here in an introductory manner due to the space limitations, with the understanding that a more in-depth presentation will follow in a future chapter. Her earliest work was on frog skeletal muscle, the tissue used most commonly in this field, and consisted of an exploration of intracellular ionic factors, including the effects of high energy metabolic products on the force generation of the contractile apparatus (Donaldson & Kerrick, 1975; Gordon, Godt, Donaldson, & Harris, 1973; Kerrick & Donaldson, 1972).

Because of the relevance of their findings to cardiac contractility, Donaldson and co-workers adapted the techniques for studies of mammalian ventricular contractile mechanisms. They studied the effects of various ionic changes and inotropic agents, including simulated intracellular conditions associated with ischemia and related therapies, on the force generating capability of left ventricular cells of rat and rabbit (Best, Donaldson, & Kerrick, 1977; Bond & Donaldson, 1976; Donaldson, Best, & Kerrick, 1978; Donaldson, Bond, Seeger, Niles, & Bolles, 1981; Seeger & Donaldson, 1976). These studies shed new light on the relative importance of factors such as intracellular pH and adenosine triphosphate levels in determining normal force generation, relaxation, and reversibility of alterations in force generating capability. The findings have implications for understanding effects of conditions and therapies that alter contractility and left ventricular compliance.

Donaldson and Hermansen (1978) also pursued studies related to the cellular basis of fatigue of skeletal muscle. To this end they adapted techniques developed for frog skeletal fibers for use with mammalian skeletal muscle fibers, in order that the findings would be more relevant for understanding human function. They identified a differential effect of acidosis on the various skeletal muscle fiber types that correlated with their relative fatigability. Donaldson (1984) adapted histochemical techniques for use with single cells and characterized their responses to acidosis. More recently, Donaldson (1985) focused upon the mechanism of excitation-contraction coupling in mammalian skeletal muscle fibers because this mechanism appears to be the point of failure in a type of fatigue relevant to organismal function. Knowledge of these mechanisms can serve as the basis for more clinical studies of conditions for optimum functioning of humans.

Kalbfleisch, Reinke, Porth, Ebert, and Smith (1977) studied the effect of age on circulatory performance using a 70° head-up tilt and the Valsalva maneuver. They studied two groups of normal male subjects 40 to 49 and 47 to 56 years of age and compared the results with those obtained in their previous investigation of normal male subjects 19 to 26 years old (Smith, Bonin, Wiedmeier, Kalbfleisch, & McDermott, 1974). In response to the head-up tilt, the older subjects had lower heart rate and a decline in diastolic and arterial pressure response when compared to the younger subjects. When compared between control and Phase I and control and Phase IV of the Valsalva maneuver, older subjects also had smaller heart rate increments than the younger group. The authors speculated that these differences with advancing age may have reflected altered baroreceptor sensitivity or diminished blood pressure changes associated with decreased venous compliance or increased central blood volume. The results of this study indicated that caution should be exercised in caring for older patients when they get up from bed or strain at stool following a myocardial infarct.

The following three studies were focused on the mechanism of function in response to drugs. The first drug that was examined was sodium pentobarbital, which is used commonly in the clinical setting. Cowan, Scher, and Hildebrandt (1975) studied the effects of sodium pentobarbital on the heart rate response to electrical stimulation of the right stellate ganglion of vagotomized cats. The drug significantly slowed the rise of heart rate by 20% to 30%, prolonged the decay of heart rate by 36% to 56%, and decreased the resting heart rate. One or more of the following factors may have explained the slower rise after the drug was given: delayed transmission in the postganglionic fiber (Toman, 1952), depressed release of norepinephrine from the nerve terminals, or blocking of the norepinephrine receptor sites at the heart muscle. Although the depressed resting heart rate generally has been attributed to a depression of the central sympathetic outflow, prolonged time constants of decline from this study, that is, the slower heart rate, indicated that the cause probably was an interaction with termination of norepinephrine. Investigators noted that the decreased resting heart rate in response to the drug alone could not account for the prolonged time constants of rise and decay of heart rate.

The second group of drugs that was investigated was platelet inhibitory agents such as sulfinpyrazone, aspirin, and naproxen. Davenport et al. (1981) studied the effect of platelet inhibitory doses of sulfinpyrazone and two dosages of aspirin on the collateral coronary blood flow following temporary and permanent occlusion of the left anterior descending coronary artery in anesthetized dogs. Sulfinpyrazone produced a significant increase in flow to the ischemic myocardium 5 minutes following both temporary and permanent occlusions. However, no significant increase was found in the control group or in two aspirin-treated groups.

All the drug doses significantly increased epicardial collateral flow from 5 minutes to 4 hours after permanent occlusion. Animals receiving sulfinpyrazone also demonstrated slight increase in endocardial collateral flow 4 hours after permanent occlusion, but the same was not true for the remaining groups. Although the physiologic importance of the increase in collateral flow associated with sulfinpyrazone or aspirin remained unclear, the increase may have contributed to the decreased incidence of potentially lethal arrhythmias reported after administration of either drug before acute myocardial ischemia in dogs (Moschos, Haider, Dela Cruz, Lyons, & Regan, 1978). The increase in collateral flow was insufficient to salvage myocardium. However, it may have potentiated the action of infarct-sparing drugs or enhanced delivery of beneficial drugs to ischemic myocardium and could have contributed to the reported reduction in the incidence of sudden death in patients with sulfinpyrazone after myocardial infarction (Anturane Reinfarction Trial Research Group, 1980).

Bolli, Goldstein, Davenport, and Epstein (1981) examined the potential role of platelet inhibitory agents on infarct size in anesthetized dogs with midleft anterior descending coronary artery ligation. The doses used were sufficient to inhibit adenosine diphosphate-induced platelet aggregation, and neither sulfinpyrazone nor naproxen altered infarct size. The investigators concluded that antiflammatory action, platelet inhibition, inhibition of prostaglandin synthesis, and lysosomal stabilizing activities alone do not have infarct-sparing action.

In three studies investigators dealt with an emergency procedure, cardiopulmonary resuscitation (CPR). Ralston, Babbs, and Niebauer (1982) demonstrated the effectiveness of interposed abdominal compression-CPR (IAC-CPR) in supporting circulatory function during cardiac arrest. The IAC-CPR procedure was standard CPR with abdominal compressions interposed during the release phase of chest compression. When compared with standard CPR, IAC-CPR improved arterial pressures, cardiac output, and coronary perfusion in 10 anesthetized dogs. The IAC-CPR procedure may have increased coronary flow by improving total flow and by altering favorably the distribution of aortic flow during chest recoil. Additionally, data from an electrical model of the circulation showed that IAC improved cranial and myocardial perfusion at all levels of chest compression pressure during CPR simulation, and the amount of improvement was related linearly to peak abdominal pressure (Babbs, Ralston, & Geddes, 1984).

In a subsequent study, Ralston, Voorhees, and Babbs (1984) studied the effect of intrapulmonary epinephrine instillation on blood flow to vital organs during 20 minutes of CPR and ventricular fibrillation in two groups of anesthetized dogs. Group I received no additional treatment, and Group II received intrapulmonary epinephrine instillation using a Swan Ganz catheter. In Group I, cardiac output and organ blood flow did not vary significantly. However, intrapulmonary epinephrine instillation in Group II significantly improved blood flow to the myocardium, the brain, and the adrenals, and nearly doubled the percentage of animals that were easy to resuscitate. They also demonstrated that adequate myocardial blood flow greater than 0.16 ml/min/gm was essential for initial successful resuscitation. These findings suggest that IAC-CPR and intrapulmonary epinephrine instillation might be useful in humans. However, randomized clinical trials need to precede actual implementation of these interventions.

The efficacy of nursing interventions such as pet therapy, exercise, and relaxation were examined in several studies. Baun, Bergstrom, Langston, and Thoma (1984) studied the effects of pet therapy with post infarction patients. Their study was based on suggestions made in popular and professional journals that pets may serve as a therapy in nursing homes and extended-care facilities, possibly enhancing survival rate following discharge from the coronary care unit. Data showed that both systolic and diastolic blood pressure decreased significantly over time when subjects petted a dog with whom a companion bond had been established as compared to those who petted an unknown dog. Although pet therapy per se has not been uniquely a nursing therapy, this finding may be useful for planning care for post-MI patients who enjoy having a dog and can care for it.

In both animal and human models, nurse investigators studied the effects of long-term exercise training on the cardiovascular system. Fuller and her colleagues (Owens, Fuller, Nutter, & DiGirolamo, 1977) examined the effect of a program of 12 weeks of moderate treadmill exercises in rats and found no changes, compared to a sedentary group, in body weight, food consumption, or weight of liver, kidney, spleen, and testes. They found, however, that adipose metabolism was altered by the exercise training. Fuller and Nutter (1981) also used rats to study the effects of treadmill exercises on the heart in both isolated perfused heart and intact in situ heart preparations. They reported that graded treadmill exercises failed to increase absolute ventricular mass, alter ventricular compliance, enhance nonstressed cardiac performance, or augment left ventricular reserve capacity under a range of preload conditions or in response to hypoxia. Furthermore, 12 weeks of treadmill exercises failed to change left ventricular fiber diameters, myocardial RNA, DNA, or collagen content (Nutter, Priest, & Fuller, 1981). It did, however, increase heart-weight to body-weight ratios. These changes were reversed with detraining. These data suggested that moderate levels of endurance training altered the metabolism of adipocytes but did not improve the mechanical performance of the isolated heart.

In a randomized clinical study, Sivarajan et al. (1981) studied the effects of early supervised exercises in preventing deconditioning after an acute myocardial infarction. Patients were assigned randomly to a control group or an exercise group. In-hospital exercise sessions were held for the exercise group, whereas no such formal sessions were offered to the control group. No differences between the two groups were found in clinical, hemodynamic, or electrocardiographic responses to the treadmill test. Authors also noted that the exercises were neither beneficial nor deleterious to the patients.

McCarthy (1975) and Hathaway and Geden (1983) investigated the energy expenditure involved with range of motion exercises that are commonly administered by nurses. Among normal young female volunteers, McCarthy found that active leg exercises required more energy than all other range of motion activities. Energy expenditure for all activities was related significantly to heart rate and a rating of perceived exertion. She also showed that nursing assistance supplied approximately one-half of the energy required for the unassisted exercise, and the use of active range of motion increased tidal volume 100 to 400 ml per respiration. Hathaway and Geden, on the other hand, showed that oxygen consumption and heart rate during isometric and active leg exercise programs were similar in healthy female and male subjects, but these exercises were significantly more demanding than either the passive exercise or rest program. Such studies could be an excellent guide for making nursing judgments in caring for patients who need passive or active range of motion exercises. The respiratory calorimetry used in McCarthy's study may be a viable measurement device for researchers who are pursuing similar studies.

Progressive muscle relaxation was used as a form of nursing therapy for patients with primary hypertension in a study by Pender (1984). Patients with systolic pressure above 140 mmHg or diastolic pressure above 90 mmHg were studied. The treatment group received group relaxation training followed by individual monitoring sessions over a 6-week period, but the control group did not receive relaxation training. At a 4-month follow-up, the treatment group had significantly lower mean systolic pressures than the control group. However, the difference in diastolic pressure between treatment and control groups was not significant. Judging from the moderately high inverse correlation between frequency of practice and systolic pressure at follow-up, continuous regular use of relaxation procedures appeared to be an important intervention for effective hypertension management.

Diverse studies about the cardiovascular system demonstrate nurses' vast interests and expertise. As basic mechanisms of cardiovascular function are elucidated by these nurse investigators, the theoretical base for nursing interventions will be enlarged and solidified for further expansion of nursing science. Randomized clinical trials with larger sample sizes will be necessary for most clinical studies to be recommended for application. It is encouraging, however, to note the serious attempts made by these nurse investigators in studying clinical problems that are laden with confounding variables.

GASTROINTESTINAL SYSTEM

The major cluster of studies about the gastrointestinal system was done by Walike-Hansen and her colleagues, who have contributed extensively to research in physiologic and clinical problems of the gastrointestinal area. Only a description of her research program is included here because the work will be addressed in a future chapter. Her research ranges from assessment of obesity in monkeys (Walike, B. C., Goodner, Koerker, Chideckel, & Kalnasy, 1977) and designing a liquid-diet feeding system for use with primates (Walike, B. C., Campbell, & Hillmann, 1971) to multiple studies of the regulation of food intake and factors associated with nasogastric tube feeding and parenteral nutrition. Under the general area of regulation of food intake, Walike-Hansen and her colleagues investigated the role of blood-borne substances such as glucose, insulin, glucagon, and cholecystokinin in controlling and feeding, starvation, anorexia, obesity, and satiety both in monkeys and in humans (Goodner et al., 1977; Hansen et al., 1981; Hansen, Jen, Koerker, Goodner, & Wolfe, 1982;

Hansen, Jen, Pek, & Wolfe, 1982; Koerker, Goodner, Walike-Hansen, Brown, & Rubenstein, 1978; Metzger & Hansen, 1983; Walike, B. C., 1973; Walike, B. C. & Smith, 1972). Regulation of food intake was studied also by examining the effects of caloric dilution (Hansen, Jen, & Kribbs, 1981) and meal patterns (Hansen, Jen, & Kalnasy, 1981) in monkeys. In addition, Hansen and other investigators studied the effect of somatostatin on gastric motility and meal absorption (Koerker & Hansen, 1981) and somatostatin-like immunoreactivity (SCI) on nutritional balance (Hansen, Vinik, Jen, & Schielke, 1982), as well as the role of plasma catecholamines in synchronous oscillations in plasma levels of insulin, C-peptide, glucagon, and glucose (Hansen, Schielke, et al., 1982).

Walike and colleagues also studied factors associated with nasogastric tube feeding, including lactose intolerance (Walike, B. C., & Walike, J. W., 1973, 1977), subjective distress (Padilla et al., 1979), distress reduction (Padilla et al., 1981), and temperature of tube feeding (Williams & Walike, B. C., 1975). Factors associated with parenteral nutrition such as appetite (DeSomery & Walike-Hansen, 1978; Walike-Hansen, DeSomery, Kribbs Hagedorn, & Kalnasy, 1977), diet temperature (Kagawa-Busby, Heitkemper, Hansen, Hanson, & Vanderburg, 1980), food intake and gastric motility (Martyn, Hansen, & Jen, 1984), and gastric relaxation (Heitkemper & Hansen, 1984) were also investigated by Walike-Hansen and her research team. Their contribution to the literature and the implications of findings from their research for nursing practice have been significant. Commendably, the investigators maintained both clinical and basic science perspectives in most of these studies. Readers are urged to read the primary sources.

RESPIRATORY SYSTEM

Studies of the respiratory system basically fell into two categories, the mechanism of function and treatment modalities. In the area of the mechanism of function, Kim and her coinvestigators (Kim, Druz, Danon, Machnach, & Sharp, 1976) have studied the mechanical function of the diaphragm, the principal inspiratory muscle. With anesthetized dogs, they demonstrated that the length–tension relationship of the diaphragm contributed more to the function of this muscle than did its geometry. They also found that the effective length of the diaphragm was greater than other mammalian skeletal muscles, and that the transdiaphragmatic pressure was related directly and linearly to tangential diaphragmatic tension. Their findings may have the following clinical applications: the diaphragm of severe emphysematous patients with high lung volumes (thus, shorter diaphragm length) may be able to generate appreciable force for ventilation; and transdiaphragmatic pressure (i.e., diaphragmatic force) measured in the clinical setting is a valid index of the diaphragmatic tension.

In another study, Kim, Druz, Danon, Machnach, and Sharp (1978) examined the effects of lung volume and electrode position on the electromyogram (EMG) of the diaphragm in anesthetized dogs. In a fixed thoraco-abdominal position, lung volumes were used as indicators of diaphragm muscle lengths with the diaphragmatic EMG as an index of neural output from the respiratory centers. Respiratory muscle fatigue, which usually is measured in humans by an esophageal electrode, was evaluated by using the diaphragmatic EMG. The results showed that lung volume change had little effect upon the directly recorded EMG. The effect of lung volume change upon the diaphragmatic EMG recorded from the esophagus was somewhat greater, and marked changes were noted with different esophageal recording sites. Maximal signals were observed at 1 cm above and 4 to 6 cm below the cardia in supine dogs and at 3 cm above the cardia in prone dogs. In general, the region close to the cardia appeared to be an optimal site to obtain the maximal signal. The findings of the study may be used as a guide to determine the optimal position of the esophageal electrode for diaphragm EMG measurement in humans.

Three major treatment modalities for patients with respiratory problems have been investigated. The first was respiratory muscle training, the second was the care of patients with tracheostomy, and the third was the care of patients with endotracheal suctioning. In the area of respiratory muscle training, Larson and Kim (1984) demonstrated the effectiveness of a month of daily exercises with an incentive spirometer resistive breathing device in patients with chronic obstructive pulmonary disease (COPD). With an alinear inspiratory resistance of 50 cm H_2O/L/sec at 1L/sec flow, patients increased respiratory muscle strength, but did not improve general exercise tolerance. The authors theorized that deterring the onset of respiratory muscle fatigue and respiratory insufficiency or failure by respiratory muscle training would improve patients' ventilation and tissue oxygenation (Kim, 1984). In the absence of a pharmacologic cure, respiratory muscle exercise programs have shown great potential for improving the activity level of patients with COPD.

Two studies were focused on the area of tracheostomy care, which has been a research area of interest to nursing for a long time. Crosby and Parsons (1974) developed a trachea model and measured in vitro pressures exerted by various tracheostomy and endotracheal tube cuffs. Four out of 6 tested tracheostomy tube cuffs sealed adequately against the trachea when pressures within them were less than 20 mmHg. Additionally, this study pointed out the importance of inflating the cuff with only a minimal amount of air to effectively seal the trachea.

Powaser et al. (1976) compared the effects of continuous cuff inflation, hourly deflation for 5 minutes, and a continuous air leak in anesthetized female dogs. They found less tracheal damage when the cuff had a continuous leak, but a constant tidal volume could not be maintained with this technique. There was no difference in tracheal damage between continuous cuff inflation and hourly deflation for 5 minutes. These findings emphasized the importance of using the minimum amount of air to inflate the cuff that will maintain the seal of the trachea.

Although endotracheal suctioning has been a common practice, particularly during the postoperative period, the most effective method for minimizing arterial hypoxemia has yet to be established. Naigow and Powaser (1977) compared the effects of five different suction procedures in two anesthetized dogs studied at weekly intervals for 5 weeks. The sequence of the five suction procedures was randomized. Endotracheal suctioning alone for 15 seconds produced a significant decrease in arterial oxygen tension. Arterial oxygen tension increased significantly when (a) 100% oxygen was given to spontaneously breathing dogs 3 minutes prior to suctioning, (b) lungs were hyperinflated with room air for 5 minutes following suctioning, (c) lungs were hyperinflated using 100% oxygen for 3 minutes prior to suctioning, and (d) lungs were hyperinflated with 100% oxygen before, during, and after suctioning. Interestingly, hyperinflation immediately after suctioning and continued for 5 minutes was as effective with room air as with 100% oxygen. However, caution should be exercised in extrapolating these statistically significant results to clinical practice. Randomized clinical trials with patients would be the next step in order to make a firm recommendation.

To study the effect of different suctioning techniques on arterial oxygen tension (PaO$_2$), Adlkofer and Powaser (1978) assessed the endotracheal suctioning procedure used for patients in a cardiovascular surgery intensive care unit. They observed that 54 of 64 patients were suctioned without receiving some form of preoxygenation. Ten patients were oxygenated before suctioning either by the "sigh" control on the ventilator or a self-inflating resuscitation bag connected to an oxygen source. There were considerable differences in the rate of fall in oxygen tension during endotracheal suctioning, and the amount of fall was unpredictable on the basis of duration of suctioning alone. These data suggest that preoxygenation needs to be carried out prior to suctioning in all patients. However, the effectiveness of the preoxygenation technique needs to be evaluated further.

Mechanisms responsible for the sustained fall in arterial oxygen tension after endotracheal suctioning were investigated in three anesthetized dogs by Woodburne and Powaser (1980). Their data suggested that a reflex mechanism initiated by mechanical stimulation of the airways, such as the use of a suction catheter, was responsible for the sustained fall in PaO$_2$. However, the effect of the type of anesthesia on this response needs to be clarified, and further investigation is necessary to explain the physiologic mechanisms in nonanesthetized humans.

Pursuing the same topic, Skelley, Deeren, and Powaser (1980) investigated the effects of one versus three hyperinflations with 100% oxygen, first in anesthetized dogs and later in patients recovering from cardiac surgery. They showed that a maximum fall of 33 mmHg (mean) in PaO$_2$ occurred at 30 seconds after suctioning without preoxygenation. However, both methods of preoxygenation produced a marked rise in PaO$_2$ in dogs and humans.

In the absence of conclusive evidence about its therapeutic effectiveness, Langrehr, Washburn, and Guthrie (1981) evaluated the effect of oxygen insufflation on the arterial oxygen tension level, first in controlled animal experiments and then with patients recovering from cardiac surgery. Patient comparisons also were made between oxygen insufflation during suctioning and hyperinflation with 100% oxygen done prior to suctioning. They found that oxygen insufflation minimized or prevented the fall in PaO$_2$ associated with endotracheal suctioning under their experimental conditions. Oxygen insufflation was most effective when oxygen flow rates approximated the suction flow rates, when pulmonary function was less impaired, and when subjects made spontaneous ventilatory efforts during insufflation and suctioning.

Ehrhart, Hofman, and Loveland (1981) studied a similar question to that raised by Langrehr et al. (1981), but with a model of acute respiratory failure induced by oleic acid. They found that the responses of blood gases, pH, and cardiovascular measurements to suction and apnea were similar in anesthetized, paralyzed dogs. This indicated the importance of maintaining adequate oxygenation during interruption of continuous positive pressure ventilation or intermittent positive pressure ventilation for endotracheal suction or intubation. The absence of cardiac arrhythmias during the suctioning procedures in this study provided evidence that suctioning was safe.

In general, the endotracheal suctioning procedure must be individualized to meet the specific needs of each patient. The results of the clinical studies reviewed suggest that preoxygenation is a valid and essential procedure for endotracheal suctioning in order to prevent hypoxemia and that oxygenation during and after suctioning is also beneficial in maintaining the normal oxygen tension. The collaborative role that nurses play in making decisions about such therapeutic procedures is important in achieving better patient care and advancing nursing science.

NEUROLOGIC AND NEUROENDOCRINE SYSTEM

In the neurophysiologic area, Parsons and her colleagues have investigated problems resulting from closed head injury in both experimental and clinical models. Her work is presented at an introductory level due to space limitations, and a fuller treatise will follow in a future chapter. An experimental model was used to investigate systematically cellular, nerve fiber, and nerve terminal degeneration in the rat following a single or multiple concussion(s) (Parsons & Guthrie, 1981). Changes in the sleep–wake cycle of severe closed head injured patients were investigated (Parsons, Peterson, Bell, & Holley-Wilcox, 1982), and preliminary findings revealed gross disruptions within stages of sleep as well as across stages. However, as the patient improved neurologically, the sleep architecture improved concomitantly.

Using a quasi-experimental repeated measure design with patients during the first 72 hours following severe closed head injury, Parsons and colleagues (Parsons, Peard, & Page, 1985; Parsons & Shogan,

1984; Parsons & Wilson, 1984) investigated the effects of endotracheal tube suctioning with manual hyperventilation, passive position changes, and hygiene measures. Findings from these earlier studies indicated that most nursing interventions could be carried out safely in this patient population, provided the resting mean intracranial pressure was ≤ 15 mmHg and the cerebral perfusion pressure was maintained at levels > 50 mmHg.

In the neuroendocrine system, the hypothalamus–pituitary–adrenocortical (HPA) system's responses to a variety of stress and circadian rhythm have been investigated. Twelve studies were focused on stress, and two studies were focused on circadian rhythm.

It is well known that adrenocortical steroids are necessary for the maintenance of homeostasis and the resistance of an organism to stress (Ingle, 1952; Selye, 1946). Cortisol is the main adrenocortical steroid of man, and its secretion is controlled primarily by the level of circulating adrenocorticotrophic hormone (ACTH) from the pituitary gland, which in turn is controlled by the neurohormone, corticotropin releasing factor, from the hypothalamic median eminence. During stress the levels of cortisol and ACTH are elevated markedly, but the elevated levels are incapable of exerting a negative feedback effect on the controlling system. Hence, findings from most studies of the neuroendocrine response in stress and circadian rhythm can be explained by contributing factors to either the compensating mechanism or decompensated state outlined above.

In the following six articles, researchers dealt with neuroendocrine responses to a variety of stressors. The central theme of these investigations was HPA responses to different environmental stimuli, i.e., hypoxia, hyperoxia, hypercapnea, heat, cold, and positive pressure breathing.

Changes in plasma levels of steroids may be caused by changes in secretion rate, removal rate, or a combination of both. Courtney and Marotta (1972) found that the plasma removal rate of cortisol did not change following the environmental stressors of hypoxia, hyperoxia, heat, cold, and positive pressure breathing. But dexamethasone, a synthetic corticosteroid, inhibited the adrenal secretion of cortisol in response to hypoxia (Marotta, Malasanos, & Boonayathap, 1973), indicating the operation of HPA system. Furthermore, Marotta, Sithichoke, Garcy, and Yu (1976) observed that the alterations in the serotoninergic system did not affect the HPA response to hypoxia and hypercapnea, but that increasing the activity of the adrenergic system partially prevented the usual rise of plasma corticosterone levels with these stressors. This line of inquiry was pursued further by Marotta and Sithichoke (1977) and Sithichoke and Marotta (1978). They found that the HPA system was modulated by central muscarinic cholinergic inhibition and nicotinic cholinergic quiescence during the basal state and by central nicotinic cholinergic excitation and possibly muscarinic cholinergic relaxation during a stressful state. In addition, they demonstrated that a diet deficient in choline did not affect HPA activity of the nonstressed rat, but it impaired the response to stress (Sithichoke, Malasanos, & Marotta, 1978).

Operation of the HPA system is very complex, but understanding of this system is essential for clinical nursing, which often includes stress management. As nurses continue to document the mechanisms of the HPA system, they will be able to use that knowledge to design and test nursing interventions for relieving stress.

Marotta and co-workers also examined the role of the liver in determining plasma steroid levels. In rats they demonstrated a rhythmic and inverse relationship between corticosterone levels and enzyme activity in the liver (Marotta, Hiles, Lanuza, & Boonayathap, 1975). Partial hepatectomy resulted in higher levels of plasma and adrenal corticosterone during the morning peak, but slower corticosterone rise in response to hypoxic stress (Witek-Janusek, Yu, & Marotta, 1984). These investigators concluded that the liver does play an important role in the regulation of cortisol levels.

At the clinical level, research on stress included both the effects of stressors and the effects of therapeutic interventions in relieving stress. Minckley (1974) compared the effect of prolonged, indefinite waiting before surgery to early, definite scheduling of surgery in two groups of patients who had the same type of corrective hip surgery. Both physiologic and psychologic variables were used to test the effect. She found that the stress of a prolonged, indefinite preoperative waiting period on the morning of surgery did not affect patients' rate of recovery. This finding was contrary to the general expectation that an indefinite preoperative waiting period would be stressful and make the recovery from the surgery slower. This may indicate that the relationship of preoperative stress to postoperative recovery was too weak to be detected by the instruments used in this study.

Randolph (1984) observed that therapeutic touch did not alter the individual's skin conductance, electromyogram, and skin temperature responses to a stressful film. Interventions such as therapeutic touch need to be used carefully, with consideration given to individual preference, readiness, and expectations.

Such isolated studies as those just reviewed preclude any meaningful recommendations for nursing practice. However, they point to a need for good cluster studies with reasonable sample size in order to make significant impact on clinical nursing science. Findings from basic science studies and clinical observations indicate that the levels of selected plasma or urinary constituents follow a 24-hour pattern of variation and indicate humanity's adaptation to a changing environment. These circadian rhythms are of interest to nurses and other health care providers for such purposes as determining the optimum time for administering drugs, treatments, or other interventions.

Marotta and associates examined the relationship between steroids and cations by reversing the lighting schedules in rats (Marotta, Lanuza, & Hiles, 1974) and by studying healthy women at basal state, during normal sleep–wake cycles, and after one week of reversed sleep–wake cycles (Lanuza & Marotta, 1974). Results from their studies showed that the steroid levels did not play a major role in determining the level of cations such as calcium, magnesium, zinc, and copper, even though the rhythm of steroids changed with modifications in lighting patterns and sleep–wake cycles. Their findings may indicate that stress responses of nurses who work on rotating schedules are different and that rotation periods should be long enough for them to adapt to new circadian rhythms.

NEONATAL NURSING

A cluster of clinical studies in neonatal nursing is found in the area of nonnutritive sucking, that is, the use of a pacifier. Burroughs and her colleagues carried out a series of studies to determine whether or not nonnutritive sucking decreases restlessness in neonates, thereby preserving energy reserves. Their initial effort was a study to examine the effect of nonnutritive sucking on transcutaneous oxygen tension (tc-PO_2) in noncrying preterm neonates (Burroughs, Asonye, Anderson-Shanklin, & Vidyasagar, 1978). Nonnutritive sucking produced no significant change in $tcPO_2$ levels for neonates breathing room air; however, the same treatment produced a significant increase in $tcPO_2$

in neonates on assisted ventilation. These data suggested that sucking is physiologically safe and sucking facilitated more adequate oxygenation in noncrying, preterm neonates.

Measel and Anderson (1979) investigated the effect of nonnutritive sucking on premature infants during and following every tube feeding, which is a common method of feeding for preterm infants. A treatment group was offered a pacifier during and following every tube feeding, and a control group received routine care. The treatment group showed readiness for bottle feeding 3.4 days earlier than the control group, that is, with 27 fewer tube feedings each, gained 2.6 gm/day more, and were discharged 4 days sooner. This study showed that the clinical course was improved by nonnutritive sucking opportunities offered during and following tube feedings. Because it is safe, simple, inexpensive, and easy to administer, nonnutritive sucking via a pacifier may be recommended for use by premature infants.

Still in the same area, Burroughs, Anderson, Patel, and Vidyasagar (1981) examined the relationship between tcPO₂ and strength of the sucking movements in preterm infants. An electronic suckometer was used to measure the suction and expression components of the sucking response. Data showed that infants with tcPO₂ values above 50 Torr had appreciably stronger suction pressures than did those with tcPO₂ values at or below 50 Torr. Suction pressures were significantly greater for infants with a gestational age of 30 weeks or more than for infants of less than 30 weeks gestation. This study suggested that gestational age was a more reliable indicator of the sucking strength than postnatal age.

Anderson, McBride, Dahm, Ellis, and Vidyasagar (1982) investigated the development of the sucking response in 30 normal infants from 1 to 5 minutes postbirth until their first feeding, which was usually 4 hours after birth. Mothers were not given tranquilizers or analgesics during labor. Six mothers received no medication for delivery, but others received the following forms of anesthesia: paracervical nerve blocks, pudendal nerve blocks, and both a paracervical and a pudendal block. The typical medication was 2% Nesacaine for paracervical blocks and 1% Xylocaine for pudendal blocks. Mean sucking pressures were 5 Torr at birth, 103 Torr at 90 minutes, and 65 Torr at 4 hours. Those results suggested that if frequent nonnutritive sucking opportunities are provided from birth, clinically normal infants could begin feeding successfully at 1 or 2 hours postbirth instead of 4 hours after birth.

In yet another study, Ostler and Anderson-Shanklin (1979) examined the relationship between early feeding and the incidence and severity of neonatal physiologic jaundice. Ten infants (experimental group) were first fed one hour after delivery and 10 others (control group) 6 hours after birth. Infants who were offered feedings at one hour were able to take these feedings as successfully as those infants who were fed at 6 hours. The experimental group passed meconium significantly earlier and had significantly lower levels of serum bilirubin than the control group.

In summary, these five studies related to neonate sucking and feeding indicated that nonnutritive sucking improved oxygenation in preterm neonates and may have reduced the hospitalization time of premature infants when it was offered during and following tube feedings. Gestational age appeared to be a more reliable indicator of the strength of the sucking than postnatal age. When frequent nonnutritive sucking opportunities are given from birth, feeding may begin between 1 and 2 hours postbirth, rather than at 4 hours. Lastly, infants who had feeding at one hour of life passed meconium significantly earlier and had significantly lower serum bilirubin than infants who had their first feeding at the 6th hour of life. This cluster of studies pursued by one investigator and her colleagues has been an exemplary case of mentorship that deserves much emulation.

SUMMARY AND FUTURE DIRECTIONS

This review included basic science literature and nursing, clinical and research literature on physiologic responses to health and illness across the life span. The universe of knowledge generated through these studies was quite diverse, and the relevance to nursing science varied. Articles published in basic science research journals were selected when the nursing implication was evident, and these tended to fall into the category of studies of mechanism of function. These studies contributed to a theoretical underpinning for nursing in its evolution as an applied science. Although direct application of these studies to clinical practice may not be possible in all instances, they provided some scientific base for many commonly used nursing therapies. Interpretation of the results of clinical studies required caution when confounding variables were not controlled. These either should have been ruled out or controlled statistically so that the effect of nursing therapy could be associated directly with the outcome of the study. Careful attention to this particular area in future research will help establish internal validity of the research findings, thereby making nursing interventions highly specific and sensitive.

The review of these articles demonstrates clearly the need for nurses to have advanced knowledge in both physiology and biochemistry in order to grasp fully the concepts of physiologic phenomena at the cellular level. Understanding and investigation of these concepts not only will enhance the ability of nurses to provide scientific nursing therapies but also will expand the knowledge base for nursing science.

It is exciting and at the same time challenging to observe the diverse expertise of nurse physiologists and nurse researchers. The trend of nurse physiologists' research moving into the clinical arena is encouraging; however, complete amalgamation of the two is yet to come. During this stage of nursing science development, I would urge nurses and editors of nursing research journals to be receptive to the studies of basic scientists such as nurse physiologists, and nurse physiologists to be more attentive to the uniqueness of nursing as a distinct scientific discipline. More basic science articles need to be published in nursing research journals, and nurses in general need to broaden their scope of reading and publication. I believe such integration certainly will enlarge the knowledge base for nursing science. Physiology is an essential ingredient in maintaining the holistic nature of nursing science; hence, more physiologic studies should be integrated into the mainstream of nursing literature.

REFERENCES

Adlkofer, R. M., & Powaser, M. M. (1978). The effect of endotracheal suctioning on arterial blood gases in patients after cardiac surgery. *Heart & Lung, 7,* 1011–1014.

American Nurses' Association. (1980). *ANA Social Policy Statement.* Kansas City, MO: Author.

American Nurses' Association. (1984). *Directory of nurses with doctoral degrees.* Kansas City, MO: Author.

Anderson, G. C., McBride, M. R., Dahm, J., Ellis, M. K., & Vidyasagar, D. (1982). Development of sucking in term infants from birth to four hours postbirth. *Research in Nursing and Health, 5,* 21–27.

Anturane Reinfarction Trial Research Group. (1980). Sulfinpyrazone in the prevention of sudden death after myocardial infarction. *New England Journal of Medicine, 302,* 250-256.

Babbs, C. F., Ralston, S. H., & Geddes, L. A. (1984). Theoretical advantages of abdominal counterpulsation in CPR as demonstrated in a simple electrical model of the circulation. *Annals of Emergency Medicine, 13,* 660-671.

Baun, M. M., Bergstrom, N., Langston, N. F., & Thoma, L. (1984). Physiological effects of human/companion animal bonding. *Nursing Research, 33,* 126-129.

Best, R. M., Donaldson, S. K. B., & Kerrick, W. G. L. (1977). Tension in mechanically disrupted mammalian cardiac cells: Effects of magnesium adenosine triphosphate. *Journal of Physiology, 265,* 1-17.

Bolli, R., Goldstein, R. E., Davenport, N., & Epstein, S. E. (1981). Influence of sulfinpyrazone and naproxen on infarct size in the dog. *American Journal of Cardiology, 47,* 841-847.

Bond, E., & Donaldson, S. K. B. (1976). Intracellular effects of simulated ischemia on contractility of mammalian left ventricular cardiac muscle. *Communicating Nursing Research, 9,* 117-127.

Burroughs, A. K., Anderson, G. C., Patel, M. K., & Vidyasagar, D. (1981). Relation of non-nutritive sucking pressures to $tcPO_2$ and gestational age in preterm infants. *Perinatology-Neonatology, 5,* 54-62.

Burroughs, A. K., Asonye, U. O., Anderson-Shanklin, G. C., & Vidyasagar, D. (1978). The effect of non-nutritive sucking on transcutaneous oxygen tension in noncrying, preterm neonates. *Research in Nursing and Health, 1,* 69-75.

Courtney, G. A., & Marotta, S. F. (1972). Adrenocortical steroids during acute exposure to environmental stresses: I. Disappearance of infused cortisol. *Aerospace Medicine, 43,* 46-51.

Cowan, M. J., Bruce, R. A., & Reichenbach, D. D. (1984). Estimation of inferobasal myocardial infarct size by late activation abnormalities of the QRS complex. *American Journal of Cardiology, 54,* 726-732.

Cowan, M. J., Reichenbach, D. D., Bruce, R. A., & Fisher, L. (1982). Estimation of myocardial infarct size by digital computer analysis of the VCG. *Journal of Electrocardiology, 15,* 307-316.

Cowan, M. J., Scher, A. M., & Hildebrandt, J. (1975). Heart rate response to sympathetic stimulation before and after sodium pentobarbital. *American Journal of Physiology, 228,* 1568-1574.

Crosby, L. J., & Parsons, L. C. (1974). Measurements of lateral wall pressures exerted by tracheostomy and endotracheal tube cuffs. *Heart & Lung, 3,* 797-803.

Davenport, N., Goldstein, R. E., Capurro, N., Lipson, L. C., Bonow, R. O., Shulman, N. R., & Epstein, S. E. (1981). Sulfinpyrazone and aspirin increase in epicardial coronary collateral flow in dogs. *Journal of Cardiology, 47,* 848-854.

DeSomery, C. H., & Walike-Hansen, B. (1978). Regulation of appetite during total parenteral nutrition. *Nursing Research, 27,* 19-24.

Donaldson, S. K. B. (1984). Ca^{2+}-activated force generating properties of mammalian skeletal muscle fibers: Histochemically identified single peeled rabbit fibres. *Journal of Muscle Research and Cell Motility, 5,* 593-612.

Donaldson, S. K. B. (1985). Peeled mammalian skeletal muscle fibers: Possible stimulation of Ca^{2+} release via the TT-SR junction. *Journal of General Physiology, 86,* 501-525.

Donaldson, S. K. B., Best, R. M., & Kerrick, W. G. (1978). Characterization of the effects of Mg^{2+} on Ca^{2+}-activated tension generation of skinned rat cardiac fibers. *Journal of General Physiology, 71*, 645-656.

Donaldson, S., Bond, E., Seeger, L., Niles, N., & Bolles, L. (1981). Intracellular pH versus $MgATP^{2-}$ concentration: Relative importance as determinants of Ca^{2+}-activated force generation of disrupted rabbit cardiac cells. *Cardiovascular Research, 15*, 268-275.

Donaldson, S. K. B., & Hermansen, L. (1978). Differential, direct effects of H^+ on Ca^{2+}-activated force of skinned fibers from the soleus, cardiac and adductor magnus muscles of rabbits. *Pflugers Archives, 376*, 55-65.

Donaldson, S. K. B., & Kerrick, W. G. L. (1975). Characterization of the effects of Mg^{2+} on Ca^{2+}-activated tension generation of skinned skeletal muscle fibers. *Journal of General Physiology, 66*, 427-444.

Ehrhart, I. C., Hofman, W. F., & Loveland, S. R. (1981). Effects of endotracheal suction versus apnea during interruption of intermittent or continuous positive pressure ventilation. *Critical Care Medicine, 9*, 464-468.

Fuller, E. O., & Nutter, D. O. (1981). Endurance training in the rat. II. Performance of isolated and intact heart. *Journal of Applied Physiology, 51*, 941-947.

Goodner, C. J., Walike, B. C., Koerker, D. J., Ensinck, J. W., Brown, A. C., Chideckel, E. W., Palmer, J., & Kalnasy, L. (1977). Insulin, glucagon, and glucose exhibit synchronous, sustained oscillations in fasting monkeys. *Science, 195*, 177-179.

Gordon, A. M., Godt, R. E., Donaldson, S. K. B., & Harris, G. E. (1973). Tension in skinned frog muscle fibers in solutions of varying ionic strength and neutral salt composition. *Journal of General Physiology, 62*, 550-574.

Hansen, B. C., Jen, K.-L. C., & Kalnasy, L. (1981). Control of food intake and meal patterns in monkeys. *Physiology and Behavior, 27*, 803-810.

Hansen, B. C., Jen, K.-L. C., Koerker, D. J., Goodner, C. J., & Wolfe, R. A. (1982). Influence of nutritional state on periodicity in plasma insulin levels in monkeys. *American Journal of Physiology, 242*, R255-R260.

Hansen, B. C., Jen, K.-L. C., & Kribbs, P. (1981). Regulation of food intake in monkeys: Response to caloric dilution. *Physiology & Behavior, 26*, 479-486.

Hansen, B. C., Jen, K.-L. C., Pek, S. B., & Wolfe, R. A. (1982). Rapid oscillations in plasma insulin, glucagon, and glucose in obese and normal weight humans. *Journal of Clinical Endocrinology and Metabolism, 54*, 785-792.

Hansen, B. C., Pek, S., Koerker, D. J., Goodner, C. J., Wolfe, R. A., & Schielke, G. P. (1981). Neural influences on oscillations in basal plasma levels of insulin in monkeys. *American Journal of Physiology, 240*, E5-E11.

Hansen, B. C., Schielke, G. P., Jen, K.-L. C., Wolfe, R. A., Movahed, H., & Pek, S. B. (1982). Rapid fluctuations in plasma catecholamines in monkeys under undisturbed conditions. *American Journal of Physiology, 242*, E40-E46.

Hansen, B. C., Vinik, A., Jen, K.-L. C., & Schielke, G. P. (1982). Fluctuations in basal levels and effects of altered nutrition on plasma somatostatin. *American Journal of Physiology, 243*, R289-R295.

Hathaway, D., & Geden, E. A. (1983). Energy expenditure during leg exercise programs. *Nursing Research, 32*, 147-150.

Heitkemper, M., & Hansen, B. C. (1984). Gastric relaxation prior to enteral feeding. *Journal of Parenteral and Enteral Nutrition, 8*, 682-684.

Hockenberger, J. M., & Rubin, M. B. (1974). Cyclic occurrence of premature ventricular contractions in acute myocardial infarction patients: A pilot study. *Nursing Research, 23*, 489–491.

Ingle, D. J. (1952). The role of the adrenal cortex in homeostasis. *Journal of Clinical Endocrinology, 8*, 23–37.

Kagawa-Busby, K. S., Heitkemper, M. M., Hansen, B. C., Hanson, R. L., & Vanderburg, V. V. (1980). Effects of diet temperature on tolerance of enteral feedings. *Nursing Research, 29*, 276–280.

Kalbfleisch, J. H., Reinke, J. A., Porth, C. J., Ebert, T. J., & Smith, J. J. (1977). Effect of age on circulatory response to postural and valsalva tests. *Proceedings of the Society for Experimental Biology and Medicine, 156*, 100–103.

Kerrick, W. G. L., & Donaldson, S. K. B. (1972). The effect of Mg^{2+} on submaximum Ca^{2+} activated tension in skinned fibers of frog skeletal muscle. *Biochimica et Biophysica Acta, 275*, 117–122.

Kim, M. J. (1984). Respiratory muscle training: Implications for patient care. *Heart and Lung, 13*, 333–339.

Kim, M. J., Druz, W. S., Danon, J., Machnach, W., & Sharp, J. T. (1976). Mechanics of the canine diaphragm. *Journal of Applied Physiology, 41*, 369–382.

Kim, M. J., Druz, W. S., Danon, J., Machnach, W., & Sharp, J. T. (1978). Effects of lung volume and electrode position on the esophageal diaphragmatic EMG. *Journal of Applied Physiology, 45*, 392–398.

Koerker, D. J., Goodner, C. J., Walike-Hansen, B., Brown, A. C., & Rubenstein, A. H. (1978). Synchronous, sustained oscillation of C-peptide and insulin in the plasma of fasting monkeys. *Endocrinology, 102*, 1649–1652.

Koerker, D. J., & Hansen, B. C. (1981). Influence of somatostatin on gastric motility and meal absorption in rhesus monkeys, (*Macaca mulatta*). *Metabolism, 30*, 335–339.

Langrehr, E. A., Washburn, S. C., & Guthrie, M. P. (1981). Oxygen insufflation during endotracheal suctioning. *Heart & Lung, 10*, 1028–1036.

Lanuza, D. M., & Marotta, S. F. (1974). Circadian and basal interrelationships of plasma cortisol and cations in women. *Aerospace Medical Association, 45*, 864–868.

Larson, M., & Kim, M. J. (1984). Respiratory muscle training with the incentive spirometer resistive breathing device. *Heart & Lung, 13*, 341–345.

Lindsey, A. (1982). Phenomena and physiological variables of relevance to nursing, review of a decade of work: Part I. *Western Journal of Nursing Research, 4*, 343–364.

Lindsey, A. (1983). Phenomena and physiological variables of relevance to nursing, review of a decade of work: Part II. *Western Journal of Nursing Research, 5*, 41–63.

Lindsey, A. (1984). Research for clinical practice: Physiological phenomena. *Heart & Lung, 13*, 496–506.

Marotta, S. F., Hiles, L. G., Lanuza, D. M., & Boonayathap, U. (1975). The relation of hepatic in vitro inactivation of corticosteroids to the circadian rhythm of plasma corticosterone. *Hormone and Metabolic Research, 7*, 334–337.

Marotta, S. F., Lanuza, D. M., & Hiles, L. G. (1974). Diurnal variations in plasma corticosterone and cations of male rats on two lighting schedules. *Hormone and Metabolic Research, 6*, 329–331.

Marotta, S. F., Malasanos, L. J., & Boonayathap, U. (1973). Inhibition of the adrenocortical response to hypoxia by dexamethasone. *Aerospace Medicine, 44*, 1-4.

Marotta, S. F., & Sithichoke, N. (1977). Actions of cholinergic agonist and antagonists on the adrenocortical response of basal, hypoxic, and hypercapnic rats. *Aviation, Space and Environmental Medicine, 48*, 446-450.

Marotta, S. F., Sithichoke, N., Garcy, A. M., & Yu, M. (1976). Adrenocortical responses of rats to acute hypoxic and hypercapnic stresses after treatment with aminergic agents. *Neuroendocrinology, 20*, 182-192.

Martyn, P. A., Hansen, B. C., & Jen, K.-L. C. (1984). The effects of food intake and gastric motility. *Nursing Research, 33*, 336-342.

McCarthy, R. T. (1975). Heart rate, perceived exertion, and energy expenditure during range of motion exercise of the extremities: A nursing assessment. *Military Medicine, 140*, 9-16.

Measel, C. P., & Anderson, G. C. (1979). Non-nutritive sucking during the tube feedings: Effect on clinical course in premature infants. *Journal of Obstetric, Gynecological and Neonatal Nursing, 8*, 265-272.

Metzger, B. L., & Hansen, B. C. (1983). Cholecystokinin effects on feeding, glucose, and pancreatic hormones in rhesus monkeys. *Physiology and Behavior, 30*, 509-518.

Minckley, B. B. (1974). Physiologic and psychologic responses of elective surgical patients. *Nursing Research, 23*, 392-401.

Moschos, C. B., Haider, B., Dela Cruz, C., Lyons, M. M., & Regan, T. J. (1978). Antiarrhythmic effects of aspirin during nonthrombotic coronary occlusion. *Circulation, 57*, 681-684.

Naigow, D., & Powaser, M. M. (1977). The effect of different endotracheal suction procedures on arterial blood gases in a controlled experimental model. *Heart & Lung, 6*, 808-816.

Nutter, D. O., Priest, R. E., & Fuller, E. O. (1981). Endurance training in the rat. I. Myocardial mechanics and biochemistry. *Journal of Applied Physiology, 51*, 934-940.

Ostler, C. W., & Anderson-Shanklin, G. (1979). Initial feeding time of newborn infants. Effects upon first meconium passage and serum indirect bilirubin levels. *Quarterly Pediatrics Bulletin, 6*, 63-79.

Owens, J. L., Fuller, E. O., Nutter, D. O., & DiGirolamo, M. (1977). Influence of moderate exercise on adipocyte metabolism and hormonal responsiveness. *Journal of Applied Physiology, 43*, 425-430.

Padilla, G. V., Grant, M. M., Rains, B. L., Hansen, B. C., Bergstrom, N., Wong, H. L., Hanson, R., & Kubo, W. (1981). Distress reduction and the effects of preparatory teaching films and patient control. *Research in Nursing and Health, 4*, 375-387.

Padilla, G. V., Grant, M., Wong, H., Hansen, B. W., Hanson, R. L., Bergstrom, N., & Kubo, W. R. (1979). Subjective distresses of nasogastric tube feeding. *Journal of Parenteral and Enteral Nutrition, 3*, 53-57.

Parsons, L. C., & Guthrie, M. D. (1981). Nerve fiber degeneration following a single experimental cerebral concussion in the rat. *Neuroscience Letters, 24*, 199-204.

Parsons, L. C., Peard, A. L., & Page, M. C. (1985). The effects of hygiene on the cerebrovascular status of severe closed head injured persons. *Research in Nursing and Health, 8*, 173-181.

Parsons, L. C., Peterson, P. J., Bell, S., & Holley-Wilcox, P. (1982). Electrophysiologic assessment of the comatose closed head injured patient. *Proceedings of Fifth Eastern Conference on Nursing Research, 5*, 41–47.

Parsons, L. C., & Shogan, J. S. O. (1984). The effects of the endotracheal tube suctioning/manual hyperventilation procedure on patients with severe closed head injuries. *Heart & Lung, 13*, 372–380.

Parsons, L. C., & Wilson, M. M. (1984). Cerebrovascular status of severe closed head injured patients following passive position changes. *Nursing Research, 33*(2), 68–75.

Pender, N. J. (1984). Physiologic responses of clients with essential hypertension to progressive muscle relaxation training. *Research in Nursing and Health, 7*, 197–203.

Powaser, M. M., Brown, M. C., Chezem, J., Woodburne, C. R., Rogenes, P., & Hanson, B. (1976). The effectiveness of hourly cuff deflation in minimizing tracheal damage. *Heart & Lung, 5*, 734–740.

Ralston, S. H., Babbs, C. F., & Niebauer, M. J. (1982). Cardiopulmonary resuscitation with interposed abdominal compression in dogs. *Anesthesia and Analgesia, 61*, 645–651.

Ralston, S. H., Voorhees, W. D., & Babbs, C. F. (1984). Intrapulmonary epinephrine during prolonged cardiopulmonary resuscitation: Improved regional blood flow and resuscitation in dogs. *Annals of Emergency Medicine, 13*, 79–86.

Randolph, G. L. (1984). Therapeutic and physical touch: Physiological response to stressful stimuli. *Nursing Research, 33*, 33–36.

Seeger, L., & Donaldson, S. K. B. (1976). The effects of intracellular alkalosis on mammalian cardiac contractility. *Communicating Nursing Research, 9*, 128–134.

Selye, H. (1946). The general adaptation syndrome and the diseases of adaptation. *Journal of Clinical Endocrinology, 6*, 117–230.

Sithichoke, N., Malasanos, L. J., & Marotta, S. F. (1978). Cholinergic influences on hypothalamic–pituitary–adrenocortical activity of stressed rats: An approach utilizing choline deficient diets. *Acta Endocrinologica, 89*, 737–743.

Sithichoke, N., & Marotta, S. F. (1978). Cholinergic influences on hypothalamic–pituitary–adrenocortical activity of stressed rats: An approach utilizing agonists and antagonists. *Acta Endocrinologica, 89*, 726–736.

Sivarajan, E. S., Bruce, R. A., Almes, M. J., Green, B., Belanger, L., Lindskog, B. D., Newton, K. M., & Mansfield, L. W. (1981). In hospital exercise after myocardial infarction does not improve treadmill performance. *New England Journal of Medicine, 305*, 357–362.

Skelley, B. F., Deeren, S. M., & Powaser, M. M. (1980). The effectiveness of two preoxygenation methods to prevent endotracheal suction-induced hypoxemia. *Heart & Lung, 9*, 316–323.

Smith, J. J., Bonin, M. L., Wiedmeier, V. T., Kalbfleisch, J. H., & McDermott, D. J. (1974). Cardiovascular response of young men to diverse stresses. *Aerospace Medicine, 45*, 583–590.

Toman, J. E. P. (1952). Neuropharmacology of peripheral nerve. *Pharmacological Reviews, 4*, 168–218.

Walike, B. C. (1973). A physiological and behavioral approach to understanding the mechanisms of obesity and anorexia. *Communicating Nursing Research, 6*, 201–214.

Walike, B. C., Campbell, D. J., & Hillmann, R. A. (1971). New liquid-diet feeder for primates. *Journal of Applied Physiology, 31*, 946–947.

Walike, B. C., Goodner, C. J., Koerker, D. J., Chideckel, E. W., & Kalnasy, L. W. (1977). Assessment of obesity in pigtailed monkeys (*Macaca nemistrina*). *Journal of Medical Primatology, 6*, 151–162.

Walike, B. C., & Smith, O. A. (1972). Regulation of food intake during intermittent and continuous cross circulation in monkeys (*Macaca mulatta*). *Journal of Comparative and Physiological Psychology, 80*, 372–381.

Walike, B. C., & Walike, J. W. (1973). Lactose content of tube feeding diets as a cause of diarrhea. *The Laryngoscope, 83*, 1109–1115.

Walike, B. C., & Walike, J. W. (1977). Relative lactose intolerance, a clinical study of tube-fed patients. *Journal of the American Medical Association, 238*, 948–951.

Walike-Hansen, B., DeSomery, C. H., Kribbs Hagedorn, P., & Kalnasy, L. W. (1977). Effects of enteral and parenteral nutrition on appetite in monkeys. *The Journal of Parenteral and Enteral Nutrition, 1*, 83–88.

Williams, K. R., & Walike, B. C. (1975). Effect of the temperature of tube feeding on gastric motility in monkeys. *Nursing Research, 24*, 4–9.

Witek-Janusek, L., Yu, M., & Marotta, S. F. (1984). Hypoxic and nyctohemeral responses by the adrenal cortex of partially hepatectomized rats. *Aviation, Space, and Environmental Medicine, 55*, 538–541.

Woodburne, C. R., & Powaser, M. M. (1980). Mechanisms responsible for the sustained fall in arterial oxygen tension after endotracheal suctioning in dogs. *Nursing Research, 29*, 312–316.

PART II

Research on Nursing Care Delivery

Chapter 5

Critical Care Nursing

KATHLEEN DRACUP

SCHOOL OF NURSING

UNIVERSITY OF CALIFORNIA-LOS ANGELES

CONTENTS

In this chapter a review of recent research pertinent to the delivery of nursing care in the intensive care unit (ICU) is presented. The review includes only empirical investigations reported between 1975 and 1985, with the exception of a few studies cited for historical interest. The rationale for the 10-year time period is twofold. First, a remarkable number of changes took place in the architectural design and physical environment of the ICU between 1970 and 1975. The early, makeshift units of the 1960s were replaced in most hospitals by second generation units specifically designed for the care of the critically ill (Kornfeld, 1980). Second, recent major advances in both clinical therapeutics and technology have affected dramatically our ability to sustain physiological life (Civetta, 1981). Most of the high technology equipment currently used by ICU nurses was not available 10 years ago or was limited to primitive prototypes. Given the changes in the

ICU environment and treatment modalities, a review limited to the past decade was judged the most effective means to identify pertinent questions and gaps in knowledge relevant to the practice of critical care nursing today.

The review was accomplished by computer searches that were augmented by manual searches in *Index Medicus*, the *Cumulative Index to Nursing and Allied Health Literature*, and the *International Nursing Index* and searches of individual references. The computer-aided search revealed that investigators from many disciplines besides nursing conducted research pertinent to the delivery of critical care nursing during the period under review. Moreover, they reported their findings almost exclusively in the medical and nursing literature, regardless of their professional affiliation. Therefore, all studies reported in the English language nursing or medical literature that pertained to some aspect of the delivery of critical care nursing were included. Two areas were excluded from review: research related to specific clinical nursing practice in the ICU, and studies in which various educational programs used to prepare ICU nurses for specialty practice were evaluated.

The organization of the chapter reflects the categories used for analysis of all retrieved studies. These categories were suggested inductively through the search process: (a) issues related to the delivery and evaluation of critical care nursing, including those related to the structure of the ICU, the process of nursing care, and outcome measurement; and (b) ethical dilemmas experienced by critical care nurses.

ISSUES RELATED TO THE DELIVERY OF CRITICAL CARE NURSING

Structure of Critical Care Units

ICUs traditionally have been considered stressful environments for patients, families, and staff. The stress experienced by all three groups is related to the physical structure of the unit and the policies and procedures that govern activities in an ICU, as well as to the uncertainty and loss that usually accompanies a catastrophic illness.

Impact on Patients. The research on the stress experienced by patients hospitalized in an ICU can be divided into two categories according to the methodology employed. First, researchers used descriptive designs to identify the sources of patient stress and examine the relationship between patient or unit characteristics and stress. Second, they conducted experimental studies to evaluate the effect of various nursing interventions on patient stress.

Using a retrospective design, researchers asked patients to identify significant stressors during their hospitalization in the ICU (Davis, 1978; Geertsen, Ford, & Castle, 1976; Jones, Withey, & Ellis, 1979; Meffert et al., 1980; Nastasy, 1985; Patacky, Garvin, & Schwirian, 1985; Riggio, Singer, Hartman, & Sneider, 1982). Despite the impressive heterogeneity among the patient samples, the majority of investigators reported similar sources of stress: noise, lack of sleep, social isolation, enforced immobility, pain from procedures, and poor communication with staff.

One descriptive study was performed specifically to identify noise levels in the ICU setting (Redding, Hargest, & Minsky, 1977). Using wall microphones placed two feet above the patient's head, the investigators documented noise levels above 70 decibels (dB) that were consistent throughout the 24 hours and that exceeded the limits set by the International Noise Council of 45 dB for day, 40 dB for evening, and 20 dB for nights (Hansell, 1984).

Noble (1979) studied staff communication and found that only 14% took place with the patient, whereas the remainder was among staff, particularly the nurses. In addition, the researcher found that conversations that took place at the patient's bedside were largely of a personal nature. Based on these findings, both Noble and Redding et al. (1977) recommended that new ICUs be built to include staff conference rooms and additional insulation in high noise level areas, for example, nursing stations and utility rooms. The effects of such architectural modifications remain untested.

The restriction of visitors in the ICU was addressed by only one investigator. Kirchoff (1982) conducted a national survey of coronary care units (CCUs) to determine the policies related to the regulation of visiting hours. The study's strengths included careful randomization procedures and a large sample size. Kirchoff found that the majority of hospitals used structured, limited visiting hours (i.e., 10 minutes every hour for immediate family only) to control patient visitation. No information is currently available about visitation policies in other types of critical care units, nor has the relationship between limited visiting regulations and the patients' reported sense of isolation been established.

A number of comparative or correlational studies were conducted to identify the environmental characteristics of the typical ICU. The first-generation units were, for the most part, converted open wards that offered little privacy or quiet. As the makeshift settings gave way to units designed specifically for the care of the acutely ill patient, the frequent incidence of psychiatric disturbance documented in postcardiac surgical patients in early studies (Blachly & Starr, 1964; Egerton & Kay, 1964; Kornfeld, Zimberg, & Malm, 1965) led to new architectural designs. These included private cubicles with draped glass partitions for privacy, windows, clocks, and central monitors. These changes were designed to maintain day–night patterns of lighting, to reduce noise, and to eliminate the viewing by patients and families of procedures (such as resuscitation efforts) on other patients hospitalized in the ICU.

First- and second-generation units were compared in three studies, with researchers using reported anxiety and heart rate as indicators of stress (Leigh, Hofer, & Cooper, 1972; Sczekalla, 1973; Vanson, Katz, & Krekeler, 1980). The studies were limited by small sample size, a lack of randomization procedures, and limited measurements of the physiological effects of anxiety. Nonetheless, the results of all three suggested that the design of second-generation units reduced the amount of stress experienced by critically ill patients.

Only two research teams examined the correlation of patient characteristics and the amount of stress experienced while in the ICU. Van der Lelie, Endert, Wieling, and Dunning (1981) found that the circulatory status of patients, as determined by the extent of arrhythmias and congestive heart failure, was a more important predictor of elevated plasma noradrenaline and adrenaline than admission to the CCU. Lindquist, Jeffery, Johnson, and Haus (1985) examined the relationship of perceived personal control and stress, using an anxiety questionnaire and urinary catecholamines and cortisol to assess the stress response, in a sample of male patients admitted to a CCU with possible myocardial infarction. They found that stress decreased as perceived control increased and that patients who preferred high control experienced less stress than patients who did not.

A final mention must be made of the entire area of study surrounding the phenomena called ICU psychosis, ICU syndrome, or, in the cardiac surgical patient, postcardiotomy delirium. Prior to 1975, approximately 40 studies were conducted to identify the characteristics and predictors of this psychological state characterized by impaired orientation, memory, intellectual function, and judgment (see Kornfeld, 1980, and Lasater & Grisanti, 1975, for reviews on this topic). Given the complexity of the variables operating for the critically ill patient, it proved to be extremely difficult to isolate causative and associated factors. Moreover, investigators and clinicians used a wide variety of tools to measure the syndrome (e.g., mental status exams, observational checklists, written questionnaires, and unstructured interviews), which resulted in significant variance in the documentation of the incidence. The reported incidence varied from 1% on a general CCU (Layne & Yudofsky, 1971) to 72% in a thoracic surgical unit (Sadler, 1979). Since 1975, only three studies have been reported in this area; two were methodological studies of structured interviews used to measure postcardiotomy delirium (Kotecki, 1982; Sadler, 1979). The third was an experimental study and will be discussed in the next section.

The second category of ICU patient stress research consisted of eight studies where one or more nursing interventions were evaluated in the ICU to reduce the patient stress response. Four of the eight studies included measurement of the effect of family involvement in the ICU on patient stress. Brown (1976) documented an increase in systolic blood pressure and heart rate during the first two 10-minute visits with family members after patient admission to a CCU. Fuller and Foster (1982) compared patient stress responses to three types of patient interactions: family/patient; nurse/patient when the nurse was performing a patient care task; and nurse/patient when the nurse was conversing with the patient. Their findings suggested no change in cardiovascular parameters and decreased vocal stress during family visits.

The difference in findings between the two studies can be explained by the methodological flaws present in the Brown (1976) study. Fuller and Foster (1982) used family visits on a nonadmission day, when anxiety could be expected to have stabilized, and automated monitoring devices. In contrast, Brown did not exclude the first day and used equipment that required measurement at the bedside by one of the investigators, a method that may have biased the physiological parameters measured.

Positive effects were reported on patients' state anxiety (Doerr & Jones, 1979) and the behavioral manifestations of postcardiotomy psychosis (Chatham, 1978) when nursing staff prepared families for ICU visitation. The positive results that were documented in both studies suggested that future research is warranted to evaluate various levels of family involvement in the ICU.

Only four experimental studies were conducted to evaluate the effectiveness of various nursing strategies to reduce patient stress in the ICU. The first was a study by Kallio (1982), who examined the effects of providing ICU patients with increased personal control, using fatigue, anxiety, and depression as outcome measures. Although the investigator did not control for potential intervening variables, such as medical diagnosis or premorbid personality traits, the design did include a placebo control group. The differences were not significant, but were in the predicted direction, suggesting that control-oriented interventions may be a fruitful area for future study.

Preparation for transfer from the ICU was evaluated in studies by Schwartz and Brenner (1979) and Toth (1980). The former compared two experimental groups who received structured information about transfer from the ICU to a control group. In one of the experimental groups the patients received the transfer information, whereas in the other the family members were targeted. In both experimental groups, the subjects had reduced blood pressure and heart rate on the day of transfer, fewer cardiovascular complications up to 72 hours after transfer, and experienced less stress than control patients, but few of these differences were statistically significant. Toth reported that cardiac patients who received structured preparation for transfer had lower heart rates and systolic blood pressures than a control group, although there were no significant differences in self-reported anxiety scores between treatment groups. Given the small sample sizes involved and that both transfer studies were conducted in coronary care units, these studies should be replicated using large noncoronary care samples.

A final experimental trial was reported by Hoffman, Donckers, and Hauser (1978), with a 30-minute inservice class for CCU staff serving as the independent variable. The instructor emphasized sources of stress experienced by ICU patients, and nurses were asked to formulate nursing interventions directed toward the reduction of patient stress. A comparison of self-reported patient stress before and after the educational class indicated a significant decrease in the stress levels reported by the patients following the experimental intervention. These results are limited by lack of randomization of subjects, a single setting, and an investigator-generated interview tool.

Given the assumption that the ICU setting is unnecessarily stressful for patients, the paucity of experimental studies was particularly disturbing. All but one of the studies involved a sample size of 30 or less, with multiple dependent measures. Also, all but one was conducted in an adult CCU. To date, none has been replicated. Of greatest concern was the atheoretical nature of all the research in the area of patient stress. There was little or no attempt to explore relationships among the variables by hypothesis testing with the goal of prediction, and few studies were conducted to evaluate nursing interventions directed toward stress reduction. Future work in this area is needed to delineate the relationships among personality characteristics, sociocultural factors, and physiological state in the stress experience of acutely ill patients. Psychological and environmental stressors, which have been considered interchangeable by many researchers, need to be distinguished. Finally, the results of nursing interventions to reduce patient stress need to be evaluated systematically in controlled trials using a variety of ICU patient populations.

Impact on Families.   Nine studies were performed in the area of family stress in the ICU. The dearth of intervention studies is particularly dramatic in this area, with only one of the nine using an experimental design. All eight of the descriptive studies had as their purpose to identify the families' perceived needs related to the hospitalization of their relative in the ICU, with one investigator (Prowse, 1984) also examining the extent of agreement between family members' and nurses' perceptions about nursing's responsibility to meet the identified needs. The perceived needs were ranked using a structured interview (Daley, 1984; Molter, 1979; Prowse, 1984; Rogers, 1983; Stillwell, 1984), Q sort (Bouman, 1984), or paper and pencil questionnaire with a Likert scale (Carter, Miles, Buford, & Hassanein, 1985). Despite the variation in study populations and methodologies, the reported needs were relatively consistent across studies; for example, need for hope, need for communication with staff about the patient's condition, and need for freedom of access to the patient. Although some discrepancy existed in whether cognitive needs or emotional needs were considered more important by families, these differences were minimal and probably had little clinical significance.

Unlike the nursing research on patient stress in ICUs, the investigators of family stress used a wide variety of settings, including the pediatric ICU (Carter et al., 1985) and the general adult medical–surgical ICU (Molter, 1979), as well as larger sample sizes ranging from 30 to 165. Two of the studies were focused on specific needs identified by previous investigators, namely, the need to be with the patient (Stillwell, 1984) and the need to participate in the physical care of the patient (Coppin, 1985). Stillwell confirmed the findings of earlier researchers that the majority of family members desired unrestricted visiting in the ICU, while Coppin's work revealed that the family members most likely to participate in the physical care of the patient were those who reported high trait anxiety.

Only one study was conducted to test nursing interventions directed toward meeting the needs of families in the ICU. Breu and Dracup (1978) described a set of interventions for spouses of acutely ill cardiac patients that included frequent communication between staff and family, primary nursing, unrestricted visiting for family members, and family participation in the physical care of the patient. Although their results indicated a significant difference between control and experimental family members in terms of needs met (Dracup & Breu, 1978), their study was limited by small sample size, a single setting, and multiple independent variables.

In summary, the investigators who delineated the types of stressors operating for the families of patients hospitalized in the ICU have produced relatively consistent findings. One of the important research priorities in the area of critical care nursing delivery now lies in the testing of nursing interventions related to the structure and organization of ICUs, including policies and procedures, in regard to meeting the needs of family members. The effects of such interventions on the stress levels of families and the welfare of patients remains unknown.

Impact on Nursing Staff. The paucity of data regarding patient and family stress in the ICU has been counterbalanced by a wealth of research about the stress experienced by the ICU nurse. The contention of Cross and Kelly (1983) that the stress of nurses working in hospital settings has been "dramatically ignored" and that ICU stress is particularly deserving of attention is contradicted by the number of studies that have focused on the sources of stress for ICU nurses, the effects of stress on staff, and the coping mechanisms employed. Researchers from many disciplines have shown great interest in the stress experienced by ICU staff, with nurse researchers being in the minority of principal authors for the early investigations (Stehle, 1981).

Most of the early investigators explored the types and severity of stressors experienced by ICU staff, namely, excessive workloads, communication conflicts with physicians, lack of administrative support, the constant threat of patient death and disability, dealing with anxious families, and equipment malfunction and noise (see Stehle's 1981 review of the 13 investigations reported between 1965 and 1974).

Nine studies performed since 1974 confirmed these early findings in adult ICU settings (Bailey, Steffen, & Grout, 1980; Brubakken & Ball, 1983; Huckabay & Jagla, 1979; Martino & McIntosh, 1985; Mundt, 1985; Steffen, 1980; Warner & Lopez, 1985), as well as in neonatal (Astbury & Yu, 1982; Jacobson, 1978) and pediatric ICUs (Lester & Brower, 1981). The latter investigators addressed many of the methodological limitations related to the reliability and validity of instruments that were present in earlier research. The major stressor consistently identified across all studies was heavy workload related to inadequate staffing rather than the nature of patient care activities in the ICU, for instance, working with dying patients and anxious families.

The assumption that ICU nurses experience more stress than nurses working in other areas of the general hospital has been challenged recently by a number of investigators who documented similar or lower stress levels for ICU nurses than for nurses working in general hospital wards (Johnson, 1979; Keane, Ducette, & Adler, 1985; Martino & McIntosh, 1985; Mohl, Denny, Mote, & Coldwater, 1982). These findings were substantiated further by the research of Dear, Weisman, Alexander, and Chase (1982) and Maloney (1982), who documented higher job satisfaction and lower turnover in nurses working in adult ICUs compared to those working on general medical–surgical units. Duxbury and Thiessen (1979) reported similar findings about turnover rates in neonatal ICUs. The findings of Norbeck (1985) that ICU nurses reported significantly higher psychological distress compared to published normative data for females suggested that the stress experienced by ICU nurses indeed may have been significant, but not different in severity from that of other hospital-based nurses.

The research on ICU nursing staff stress is complicated by the fact that various researchers have used different definitions of stress and different criterion measures. Although the levels of stress experienced by critical care nurses may indeed be similar to that of other hospital-based nurses, this finding also may be the result of inconsistencies in theoretical frameworks and methodologies across studies.

Another explanation for the similarity may reside in the personality structure and coping styles of nurses attracted to different specialties. In comparing nurses in different hospital settings, Maloney and Bartz (1983) noted that ICU nurses were significantly more adventurous, more oriented toward external control, and more likely to seek challenge and novelty than nurses working in general medical–surgical units. Although this was the only study where personality characteristics were targeted for comparison, its findings have the potential of explaining why perceived or documented stress appears the same among nurses in different specialties. Differences in personalities may result in different views of what constitutes a stressor.

The role of coping strategies in reducing stress also has been considered. Two longitudinal studies (Esteban, Ballesteros, & Caballero, 1983; Gribbins & Marshall, 1982) were conducted with ICU nurses to determine if their coping strategies changed over time. Both suggested that coping strategies changed as a function of experience in the unit, with humor and the setting of priorities being strategies used by nurses as they gained more clinical experience. An encouraging trend toward the study of coping strategies specific for the unique situation of ICUs was evidenced by the work of Stone, Jebsen, Walk, and Belsham, (1984), Jacobson (1983), and Oskins (1979). Their findings revealed a negative correlation between the number of coping strategies and burnout. The results of these three studies underscored the consistently documented negative correlation between perceived stress and years of clinical experience in ICU staff.

Social support as a buffer to job-related stress was delineated by Norbeck (1985). She found a difference between married and unmarried ICU nurses in terms of what constituted effective social support, with support for work activities being more important for married staff nurses than single nurses. Social support on the part of nursing administration was addressed indirectly by Duxbury, Armstrong, Drew, and Henley (1984). They found that head nurse leadership style was related significantly to burnout and job satisfaction, with the head nurse's consideration for unit nurses' needs being the most important correlate of the latter's job satisfaction.

Given the historical interest in the stress experienced by ICU nursing staff, it was surprising that only one study was conducted to measure the effect of an intervention on staff stress (Dubovsky, Getto, Gross, & Paley, 1977). Although this investigation documented positive results from a psychiatrist-led staff support group, no further replications were reported. Once again, controlled trials to measure the often-repeated suggestions for stress reduction need to be conducted and replicated in a variety of ICU settings. Further, empirically based research on the impact of situational and personality factors on individual coping also needs to be conducted to provide support for data-based interventions.

In summary, the lack of theoretical foundations characteristic of the early research in the area of ICU staff stress was corrected in recent studies. Investigators attempted to build predictive models using hierarchical regression analyses. A major gap continues to exist in the area of stress reduction interventions for ICU nurses. Many approaches, such as 12-hour shifts and support groups, are described in the literature and even implemented in practice, but they await empirical testing.

Process of Critical Care Nursing

The delivery of nursing care in a critical care unit is inexplicably bound to the specialized environment of the ICU and the provision of medical care. The overlap between the domains of nursing and medicine is significant because of the unique demands presented by patients with catastrophic illnesses who are in physiological crisis. Therefore, it is difficult to assess the particular contributions of nursing versus medicine in critical care, a fact reflected in the paucity of studies in this area.

The first study was conducted by Cullen and colleagues (Cullen, Civetta, Briggs, & Ferrara, 1974), who devised a scoring system to measure the intensity of care delivered to the ICU patient. The Therapeutic Intervention Scoring System (TISS) included assigned weights from 0 to 4 to grade approximately 75 various therapeutic, diagnostic, and monitoring tasks. The weights reflected the amount of time each task required, as well as its complexity. The weights were added to obtain a total score that reflected the intensity of nursing care and the amount of resources being used. The system was revised in 1983 (Keane & Cullen) and has proven helpful in determining resource allocation in ICUs (Galanes, Harris, Dulski, & Chamberlin, 1986).

A national survey was conducted in 1979 by the American Association of Critical-Care Nurses (AACN) to identify the characteristics of critical care nursing practice. The potential sample for the national survey consisted of the 4,919 hospitals listed with the American Hospital Association as having one or more critical care units. Of these,

49% ($n = 2,412$) responded (Disch, 1981). This survey continues to provide the primary data on patterns of nursing practice in critical care.

The results of the survey were reported in a series of articles detailing: (a) the characteristics of hospitals with critical care units (Disch, 1981); (b) the characteristics of the units themselves (Kinney, 1981); (c) the responsibilities of the ICU nursing staff (Breu & Dracup, 1982); (d) the equipment used in the delivery of nursing care (Holmes, 1982); (e) and patterns of staffing (Sullivan & Breu, 1982). During the time of the survey, the majority of hospitals in the United States had only one ICU, a combined medical–surgical–coronary care unit. As might be expected, there was a positive correlation between the size of the institution and the number and types of units, with hospitals under 200 beds having only one multipurpose unit and hospitals over 500 beds having an average of four specialized units. As reported by Breu and Dracup (1982), the nursing staff in the reporting ICUs performed a variety of activities (e.g., intravenous drug administration, defibrillation, fluid replacement therapy, peritoneal dialysis); all but 2 of the 16 activities listed required physician's orders or standing protocols. Nursing staff in two thirds of the units conducted patient care conferences on a regular basis; staff in one third used peer review to evaluate nursing care. Nurses in 85% of the critical care units performed chart audits as a form of patient care evaluation. In general, staff nurses had little involvement in the development of written policies and procedures governing patient admission criteria, unit management, and nursing practice.

Folk-Lightly and Brennan (1979) asked 201 ICU nurses from 11 randomly selected hospitals to rank a list of 24 commonly performed activities in terms of the amount of time they engaged in the activity, its importance as a nursing function, and the required degree of professionalism. Although the activities were similar to those identified by Breu and Dracup (1982), this second study provided new insight into the value ascribed to the activities by ICU nurses. For example, the respondents ranked "taking vital signs and measuring intake and output" as the activity that required the highest amount of their time out of a possible 24 tasks; however, they ranked the same activity 5.5 (out of a possible 24) in terms of importance, and 15 (out of 24) in terms of professionalism.

All three studies were designed and conducted carefully. The researchers provided important data from multiple settings about the process of delivering nursing care in critical care units. However, these studies need to be replicated, particularly to determine if the publication and adoption of official standards of nursing care for the critically ill patient (Thierer, Perhus, & McCracken, 1981) have made a difference in the process of critical care nursing.

Outcome of Critical Care

The critically ill patient needs and receives an impressive array of nursing and medical resources. Vast amounts of money, personnel, time, space, and highly sophisticated equipment are expended to provide care and to promote recovery. Given a society with limited resources, two questions have been posed by researchers from a number of different disciplines, including nursing: First, what is the effectiveness of intensive care on patient outcome, particularly morbidity and mortality? Second, are there subsets of patients currently admitted to the ICU who do not need or benefit from intensive care?

Effectiveness of Intensive Care.   In an attempt to document the impact of intensive care on patients, some investigators compared mortality rates in the critical care units with rates among historical controls (Griner, 1972; Mulligan, 1975; Piper & Griner, 1974; Rogers, Weiler, & Ruppenthal, 1972) or with patients assigned to conventional care (Bain, Siskind, & Neilson, 1981; Parno, Teres, Lemeshow, & Brown, 1982). Given their methodological limitations, these studies did not establish that admission to an ICU resulted in improved patient outcome over conventional hospital care.

Two randomized clinical trials in England were conducted in a postmyocardial infarction population to compare the results of home treatment with treatment in an acute CCU. The first was conducted by Mather et al. (1976) and involved 1,895 male patients under 70 years of age who had suffered an acute myocardial infarction within 48 hours of study entry. The results indicated no significant advantage to treatment in an ICU. At 28 days after entry into the study, the mortality rate was 12% for the patients randomly assigned to home care and 14% for the group treated in the CCU. At 330 days the corresponding figures were 20 and 27%. Neither comparison showed differences that were statistically significant ($p > .05$). Unfortunately, significant methodological flaws compromised the study's results. Only 24% of the patients could be allocated randomly to the two treatment groups; the remainder elected treatment at home or in the hospital. The randomized group were affected further by significant crossover between the two groups. Finally, many patients were seen late after the onset of their symptoms, which possibly encouraged high-risk patients to elect hospital care and thus biased the home group toward patients with fewer complications.

In a follow-up study also conducted in England, Hill, Hamptom, and Mitchell (1978) arranged for a physician and CCU nurse to respond to 500 calls from general practitioners. Of these, 349 patients (70%) were suspected of having myocardial infarction. Twenty-four percent of the 349 patients were excluded from the study based on predetermined medical and social criteria. The remaining 264 patients (76%) were randomized into either hospital or home treatment groups. Analysis of the nonrandomized patients revealed a high risk group that were identified appropriately by the physician–nurse team as requiring hospitalization. A final cohort of 150 patients (79 in the home group and 71 in the CCU group) were followed for six weeks. No significant difference in mortality existed between the home group (13%) and the ICU group (11%).

These two British studies have not been replicated, nor have similar studies been conducted in a general ICU population. Moreover, it is unlikely that any randomized trials will be conducted in the future comparing intensive care to conventional or home care. Given the resources available in a critical care unit, few physicians or nurses would consider it ethically sound to randomly assign a group of severely ill patients to conventional treatment. Thus, the ultimate question about the assumed superiority of intensive care compared to care provided in the patient's home or on a conventional hospital ward remains unanswered.

Although the two British investigations had significant limitations, the results indicated that there may be subgroups of patients who are unlikely to benefit from admission to an ICU. One of these subgroups may consist of patients who are admitted for the monitoring of potential complications, for example, uncomplicated post-myocardial infarction patients. Some investigators have reported that 50% to 77% of patients in general medical–surgical ICUs were admitted primarily for monitoring by nursing staff (Knaus, LeGall, et al., 1982; Thibault et al., 1980). They also suggested that these patients may not require intensive care. Certainly, low-risk patients should be considered for early transfer from the ICU (Mulley et al., 1980).

Prediction of Prognosis.   A second subgroup of patients identified as receiving questionable benefit from treatment in critical care units were those whose condition was so advanced that they could not survive regardless of treatment (Jennett, 1984). If such patients were identified prior to admission to an ICU they could be spared the exposure to the hazards and discomforts of invasive monitoring and to the psychological and social deprivations associated with ICUs, as well as to the inordinate expense of intensive care. The relationship among short-term prognosis as estimated by the physician on the day of a patient's admission to ICU, actual patient outcome, and cost of hospitalization was analyzed in 1,831 admissions to a medical or coronary ICU (Detsky, Stricker, Mulley, & Thibault, 1981). The results showed that the care of nonsurvivors involved significantly higher mean expenditure than did the care of survivors ($p < .01$). This finding has been corroborated in every investigation on the topic of resource expenditure and survival in ICUs (Chassin, 1982; Cullen, Ferrara, Briggs, Walker, & Gilbert, 1976; Cullen et al., 1984; Davis, Lefrak, Miller, & Malt, 1980; Jackson, 1984). Detsky et al. (1981) went one step further and documented that the cost of ICU care for both survivors and nonsurvivors was greatest when physicians were uncertain about the patient's prognosis.

One approach used by investigators to predict prognosis in the critically ill patient has been to devise a severity of illness score based on the extent of injury and the degree of patient response. These scales have been used extensively and validated in three types of ICU patients: (a) the head trauma patient, using the Glasgow Coma Scale (Jennett & Bond, 1975; Jennett, Teasdale, Braakman, Minderhoud, & Knill-Jones, 1976); (b) the burn patient, using burn severity scales (Feller, Tholen, & Cornell, 1980); and (c) the acute myocardial infarction patient, using the Killip (Killip & Kimball, 1967) or Norris (Norris, Brandt, Caughey, Lee, & Scott, 1969) Indices.

In addition, several investigators attempted to construct severity of illness scales that would be applicable across a wide spectrum of critically ill patients. LeGall et al. (1982) used age, previous health status, and severity of acute illness as measured by the number of organ failures. Bland and Shoemaker (1985) used 28 hemodynamic and oxygen transport variables measured over time in the acutely ill surgical patient to construct a numerical index. Lemeshow and colleagues (Lemeshow, Teres, Pastides, Avrunin, & Steingrub, 1985) constructed two multiple logistic regression models using seven admission variables and seven variables reflecting treatments and patients' conditions at 24 hours following ICU admission. None of these have been subjected to the intensive testing in multiple populations required by a predictive model. Most investigators have used a retrospective design, whereas the effectiveness of any predictive model can be evaluated only prospectively.

The most extensively tested of all the indices is the Acute Physiology and Chronic Health Evaluation, called APACHE I (Knaus, Draper, et al., 1982; Knaus, LeGall, et al., 1982; Knaus, Wagner, & Draper, 1985; Knaus, Zimmerman, Wagner, Draper, & Lawrence, 1981; Scheffler, Knaus, Wagner, & Zimmerman, 1982; Wagner et al., 1984; Wagner, Knaus, & Draper, 1983), which evolved to a simpler form (APACHE II). The latter is based on age, chronic health status, and 12 physiological variables that reflect homeostasis, such as temperature, blood pressure, serum pH, and serum hematocrit (Knaus, Draper, Wagner, & Zimmerman, 1985; Wagner, Knaus, & Draper, 1986). APACHE II yields a single cardinal index number theoretically varying from 0 to 60 with an observed range of 0 to 45 (zero indicating normal physiologic balance) and an interobserver reliability of .96. Validity testing revealed stable and predictable results within a wide variety of diseases (Wagner, Knaus, & Draper, 1986). An alternate form of APACHE II was developed and tested by a team of French researchers (LeGall et al., 1984), but it awaits further validation testing.

These scales provided important and unique insights concerning the effectiveness of critical care and are useful in assuring that patients randomly assigned to various treatment groups in medical or nursing studies are indeed comparable. The APACHE II, in particular, holds exciting potential in the evaluation of critical care nursing quality, the prediction of required nurse–patient ratios, and application in clinical nursing research. As yet, this potential is untested by nurse researchers.

Prediction of Mortality. Clearly, cost containment in the ICU is served best by withholding resources from the hopelessly ill (Galanes et al., 1986), as well as transferring patients who only require anticipatory care to conventional care as soon as possible. In the past, investigators attempted to help nurses and physicians predict a patient's response to intensive medical and nursing care by detailing the natural history of specific illnesses (Fowler, Hamman, Zerbe, Benson, & Hyers, 1985; Montgomery, Stager, Carrico, & Hudson, 1985; Parno, Teres, Lemeshow, Brown, & Avrunin, 1984; Stange & Sumner, 1978; Teres, Brown, & Lemeshow, 1982) and the effects of intensive interventions (Nunn, Milledge, & Singaraya, 1979; Witek, Schachter, Dean, & Beck, 1985). Unfortunately, nurses and physicians continue to be plagued by prognostic uncertainty, a reality that is reflected painfully in the wide variety of criteria that currently exist for patients' admission to and discharge from the ICU (Teres et al., 1982).

Unfortunately, the investigators who tried to predict mortality of ICU patients fell short of their goal. First, their research suffered from significant limitations. The samples were so homogeneous, dealing with patients who had disease of a single organ system, that generalization to the usual ICU patient, with his or her unique combination of primary and secondary disease processes, therapeutic regimens, and complications of therapy and disease, was inappropriate. The majority of the researchers targeted only demographic and disease-related variables, ignoring many variables that may have had a marked effect on prognosis, such as functional status prior to admission, degree of social support, and personality and coping resources. The second reason for the failure of the predictive models lay in the extreme difficulty encountered in obtaining agreement among physicians and nurses as to what expected survival rate would be low enough to justify exclusion or withdrawal from intensive care. Unless the clinician is given a predictive mortality rate of 100%, he or she is still faced with the dilemma of recommending that lifesaving treatment be withheld from an individual patient who has the potential of recovering from an acute event. Therefore, it is not clear that any predictive model, no matter how sound methodologically, will ever address the clinician's need for certainty.

ETHICAL DILEMMAS IN CRITICAL CARE NURSING

Despite increasing interest in the area of bioethics and critical care, only five empirical studies were reported. Four of the five were focused on the problem of "do not resuscitate" orders for patients in the ICU, with two focused on the neonatal ICU staff.

Berseth, Kenny, and Durand (1984) compared the attitudes of ICU nurses and intermediate care unit nurses toward active and passive euthanasia for seriously ill infants. They found that ICU nurses were significantly less likely to favor resuscitation than were intermediate care unit nurses. Although both groups expressed the belief that the decision should be made jointly with family and staff, the ICU staff were less likely to favor resuscitation of high-risk infants than the general staff nurses.

In a related study, the compliance and noncompliance of perinatal nurses to "do not resuscitate" orders was examined by Savage, Cullen, Kirchhoff, and Pugh (1985). Peer support and the attitude of the parents were critical components in the nurses' willingness to comply with "do not resuscitate" orders policies.

Finally, patients who had been designated as "do not resuscitate" were examined in two other studies and compared with ICU patients who were not so designated in terms of demographic, physiologic, and psychosocial variables (Witte, 1984) and resources consumed, level of treatment, and survival (Lewandowski, Daly, McClish, Juknialis, & Youngner, 1985). The only three characteristics that differentiated the "do not resuscitate" patients were length of hospitalization, level of consciousness, and documentation of family wishes on the chart. Lewandowski and colleagues (1985) found no difference on any of the resource and outcome variables between patients designated "do not resuscitate" and those who were not so designated. In this latter study the investigators were the first to address the clinician's commonly expressed fear that a "do not resuscitate" order would lead to patients being abandoned by the critical care nursing staff.

A final study in the area of ethical issues was related to informed consent. Whalen (1984) performed a descriptive study to determine nurses' perspective on the disclosure of information to critically ill patients. Using the example of pulmonary artery catheter, Whalen found that nurses were more interested in describing the comforts and discomforts of the catheter insertion than its medical risks or benefits. These findings reflected nurses' concerns with patient comfort and suggested that nurses approached the subject of informed consent from a perspective that was different but complementary to physicians'.

SUMMARY

The research pertaining to the delivery of nursing care in the ICU was reviewed to describe: (a) the impact of the unit structure and organization, including policies and procedures, on patients, nurses, and families; (b) the process of critical care nursing; (c) the outcomes of critical care nursing; (d) some of the ethical issues germane to the care of the critically ill patient. Although these areas of inquiry are quite diverse, a number of similarities can be identified.

The most obvious of the similarities was that, with few exceptions, the studies pertaining to delivery of nursing care were performed by researchers from a variety of disciplines other than nursing, including medicine, psychology, public health, and economics. In many instances, such as the studies of patients' stress experiences in ICUs, these efforts enhanced our knowledge of the phenomena and complemented or replicated the efforts of nurse researchers. Unfortunately, in some areas nurse researchers were quite absent, with the result that the studies lacked a nursing perspective. For example, the large body of knowledge related to the effects of critical care on patient outcome reflected medicine's orientation toward cure.

While it is important to measure the effect of nursing care in the ICU on patient survival, the effect of nursing efforts on short- and long-term quality of life, functional status, and health maintenance is also critical and remains unknown. Nurse researchers need to build on the data base already acquired about critical care. Even more important, they need to fashion programs of research focused on the concepts central to the discipline of nursing.

A second similarity relates to the increasing quality of the reported research over the past decade. In general, early descriptive studies were conducted in a single critical care unit with a small and often biased sample. These gave way to more carefully designed, multicenter studies, although lack of randomization procedures continued to be a significant problem. Increasing attention was paid to the psychometric properties of instruments, and the validity and reliability of these instruments were appropriately discussed by the researchers using them. However, the area of family stress is a remarkable exception to this positive trend. Investigators also began to address the problem of sample homogeneity in some of the areas of inquiry by replicating their work outside the often favored CCU.

The third and final similarity lies with the preponderance of descriptive studies in all areas reviewed. Some of the data collected over the past decade can be used to build causal or predictive models. Such work can have important clinical significance, for example, in identifying patients and staff who are at risk for high stress levels in the ICU so that preventive measures might be instituted.

IMPLICATIONS AND RECOMMENDATIONS
FOR THE FUTURE

Although a large data base regarding the risks and benefits of critical care has been accumulated over the past decade, a number of avenues for future research are apparent. Much of the research to date has been atheoretical, and the data need to be reviewed, and potential conceptual schemas proposed. Future researchers should have as one of their goals the formulation and testing of appropriate theory. The work on family stress in the ICU setting provides an excellent illustration of this point. To date, only nine studies have been conducted in this area, and all shared the common goal of identifying the needs of family members in ICU. Despite the methodological limitations of the studies, the findings have been relatively consistent, both in terms of the nature of the needs and the priority each need is ascribed by family members. Nonetheless, all the studies lacked a significant theoretical base. Although such studies have the potential of providing an important proving ground for one or more of the family theories, this potential remains untried.

As with most practice specialties in nursing, there is a great need for experimental studies that evaluate the effects of various critical care nursing interventions on physical and psychosocial outcome measures. Obtaining the sample sizes required for supporting statistical tests of intervention models will continue to be a challenge and will require the cooperative efforts of nurse researchers and nurse clinicians working in multiple settings.

A final point needs to be made about research in the area of bioethics and critical care. Almost all the nursing literature in this area is theoretical in nature and lacks an empirical basis. Descriptive studies need to be performed to describe the decision-making process critical care nurses confront in the face of ethical dilemmas. Concepts such as informed consent need to be studied in the special circumstances of the ICU and elucidated through meticulously conducted descriptive research before interventions can be proposed and tested.

REFERENCES

Astbury, J., & Yu, V. Y. H. (1982). Determinants of stress for staff in a neonatal intensive care unit. *Archives of Disease in Childhood, 57*, 108–111.

Bailey, J. T., Steffen, S. M., & Grout, J. W. (1980). The stress audit: Identifying the stressors of ICU nursing. *Journal of Nursing Education, 19*(6), 15–25.

Bain, C., Siskind, V., & Neilson, F. (1981). Site of care and survival after acute myocardial infarction. *Medical Journal of Australia, 2*, 185–188.

Berseth, C. L., Kenny, J. D., & Durand, R. (1984). Newborn ethical dilemmas: Intensive care and intermediate care nursing attitudes. *Critical Care Medicine, 12*, 508–511.

Blachly, P. H., & Starr, A. (1964). Post-cardiotomy delirium. *American Journal of Psychiatry, 121*, 371–375.

Bland, R. D., & Shoemaker, W. C. (1985). Probability of survival as a prognostic and severity of illness score in critically ill surgical patients. *Critical Care Medicine, 13*, 91–95.

Bouman, C. C. (1984). Identifying priority concerns of families of ICU patients. *Dimensions of Critical Care Nursing, 3*, 313–319.

Breu, C., & Dracup, K. (1978). Helping the spouses of critically ill patients. *American Journal of Nursing, 78*, 50–53.

Breu, C., & Dracup, K. (1982). Survey of critical care nursing practice. Part III. Responsibilities of intensive care unit staff. *Heart & Lung, 11*, 157–161.

Brown, A. J. (1976). Effects of family visits on the blood pressure and heart rate of patients in the coronary care unit. *Heart & Lung, 5*, 291–296.

Brubakken, K., & Ball, M. (1983). Factors affecting job satisfaction of critical care nurses. *Heart & Lung, 12*, 430–431.

Carter, M. C., Miles, M. S., Buford, T. H., & Hassanein, R. S. (1985). Parental environmental stress in pediatric intensive care units. *Dimensions of Critical Care Nursing, 4*, 180–188.

Chassin, M. (1982). Costs and outcomes of medical intensive care. *Medical Care, 2*, 165–179.

Chatham, M. A. (1978). The effect of family involvement on patients' manifestations of postcardiotomy psychosis. *Heart & Lung, 7*, 995–999.

Civetta, J. M. (1981). Beyond technology: Intensive care in the 1980s. *Critical Care Medicine, 9*, 763–767.

Coppin, G. A. (1985). Relationship of trait anxiety to family members' participation in care of critically ill patients. *Heart & Lung, 14*, 290–291.

Cross, D. G., & Kelly, J. G. (1983). Stress and coping strategies in hospitals – A comparison of ICU and ward nurses. *The Australian Nurses Journal, 13*(2), 43–46.

Cullen, D. J., Civetta, J. M., Briggs, B. A., & Ferrara, L. C. (1974). Therapeutic intervention scoring system: A method for quantitative comparison of patient care. *Critical Care Medicine, 2*, 57–60.

Cullen, D. J., Ferrara, L. C., Briggs, B. A., Walker, P. F., & Gilbert, J. (1976). Survival hospitalization charges and follow-up results in critically ill patients. *New England Journal of Medicine, 294*, 982–987.

Cullen, D. J., Keene, R., Waternaux, C., Kunsman, J. M., Caldera, D. L., & Peterson, H. (1984). Results, charges, and benefits of intensive care for critically ill patients: Update 1983. *Critical Care Medicine, 12*, 102–106.

Daley, L. (1984). The perceived immediate needs of families with relatives in the intensive care setting. *Heart & Lung, 13*, 231–237.

Davis, B. K. (1978). The expanded measurement of patients' psychological stress responses to being in the coronary care unit. *Military Medicine, 143*, 203–207, 223–225.

Davis, H., Lefrak, S. S., Miller, D., & Malt, S. (1980). Prolonged mechanically assisted ventilation: An analysis of outcome and charges. *Journal of the American Medical Association, 243*, 43–45.

Dear, M. R., Weisman, C. S., Alexander, C. S., & Chase, G. A. (1982). The effect of the intensive care nursing role on job satisfaction and turnover. *Heart & Lung, 11*, 560–565.

Detsky, A. S., Stricker, S. C., Mulley, A. G., & Thibault, G. E. (1981). Prognosis, survival, and the expenditure of hospital resources for patients in an intensive care unit. *New England Journal of Medicine, 305*, 667–672.

Disch, J. (1981). Survey of critical care nursing practice. Part 1. Characteristics of hospitals with critical care units. *Heart & Lung, 10*, 1047–1050.

Doerr, B. C., & Jones, J. W. (1979). Effect of family preparation on the state anxiety level of the CCU patient. *Nursing Research, 218*, 315–316.

Dracup, K., & Breu, C. (1978). Using nursing research findings to meet the needs of grieving spouses. *Nursing Research, 27*, 212–216.

Dubovsky, S. L., Getto, C. J., Gross, S. A., & Paley, J. A. (1977). Impact on nursing care and mortality: Psychiatrists on the coronary care unit. *Psychosomatics, 18*, 18–27.

Duxbury, M. L., Armstrong, G. D., Drew, D. J., & Henley, S. J. (1984). Head nurse leadership style with staff nurse burnout and job satisfaction in neonatal intensive care units. *Nursing Research, 33*, 97–101.

Duxbury, M. L., & Thiessen, V. (1979). Staff nurse turnover in neonatal intensive care units. *Journal of Advanced Nursing, 4*, 591–602.

Egerton, N., & Kay, J. H. (1964). Psychological disturbances associated with open heart surgery. *British Journal of Psychiatry, 110*, 444–469.

Esteban, A., Ballesteros, P., & Caballero, J. (1983). Psychological evaluation of intensive care nurses. *Critical Care Medicine, 11*, 616–620.

Feller, I., Tholen, D., & Cornell, R. G. (1980). Improvements in burn care, 1965 to 1979. *Journal of the American Medical Association, 244*, 2074–2078.

Folk-Lightly, M., & Brennan, A. (1979). Role perception of the staff nurse in the intensive care unit. *Heart & Lung, 8*, 535–539.

Fowler, A. A., Hamman, R. F., Zerbe, G. O., Benson, K. N., & Hyers, T. M. (1985). Adult respiratory distress syndrome: Prognosis and onset. *American Review of Respiratory Disease, 132*, 472–478.

Fuller, B. F., & Foster, F. M. (1982). The effects of family/friend visits versus staff interaction on stress/arousal of surgical intensive care patients. *Heart & Lung, 11*, 457–463.

Galanes, S., Harris, B., Dulski, R., & Chamberlin, W. (1986). The I.C.U. population within the prospective payment scheme. *Heart & Lung, 15*, 515–520.

Geertsen, H. R., Ford, M., & Castle, C. H. (1976). The subjective aspects of coronary care. *Nursing Research, 25*, 211–215.

Gribbins, R. E., & Marshall, R. E. (1982). Stress and coping in the NICU staff nurse: Practical implications for change. *Critical Care Medicine, 10*, 865–867.

Griner, P. F. (1972). Treatment of acute pulmonary edema: Conventional intensive care? *Archives of Internal Medicine, 77*, 501–506.

Hansell, H. N. (1984). The behavioral effects of noise on man: The patient with "intensive care unit psychosis." *Heart & Lung, 13*, 59–65.

Hill, J. D., Hamptom, J. R., & Mitchell, J. R. A. (1978). A randomized trial of home-versus-hospital management for patients with suspected myocardial infarction. *Lancet, 1*, 837–841.

Hoffman, M., Donckers, S., & Hauser, M. (1978). The effect of nursing intervention on stress factors perceived by patients in a coronary care unit. *Heart & Lung, 7*, 804–809.

Holmes, A. (1982). Survey of critical care nursing practice. Part V. Type of equipment and responsibilities of personnel with regard to equipment. *Heart & Lung, 11*, 242–247.

Huckabay, L., & Jagla, B. (1979). Nurses' stress factors in the intensive care unit. *Journal of Nursing Administration, 9*(2), 21–26.

Jackson, B. S. (1984). A one-year mortality study of the most acutely ill patients in a medical surgical intensive care unit: Toward developing a model for selection of recipients of intensive care. *Heart & Lung, 13*, 132–137.

Jacobson, S. P. (1978). Stressful situations for neonatal intensive care nurses. *American Journal of Maternal Child Nursing, 3*, 144–150.

Jacobson, S. P. (1983). Stresses and coping strategies of neonatal intensive care unit nurses. *Research in Nursing and Health, 6*, 33–40.

Jennett, B. (1984). Inappropriate use of intensive care. *British Medical Journal, 289*, 1709–1711.

Jennett, B., & Bond, M. (1975). Assessment of outcome after severe brain damage. *Lancet, 1*, 480–484.

Jennett, B., Teasdale, G., Braakman, R., Minderhoud, J., & Knill-Jones, R. (1976). Predicting outcome in individual patients after severe head injury. *Lancet, 1*, 1031–1034.

Johnson, M. N. (1979). Anxiety/stress and the effects on disclosure between nurse and patients. *Advances in Nursing Science, 1*(4), 1–20.

Jones, B. H., Withey, K. D., & Ellis, B. W. (1979). What patients say: A study of reactions to an intensive care unit. *Intensive Care Medicine, 5*, 89–92.

Kallio, J. T. (1982). Reduction of depression: Three simple interventions. *Focus on Critical Care, 9*(4), 6.

Keane, A., & Cullen, D. (1983). Therapeutic intervention scoring system: Update 1983. *Critical Care Medicine, 11*, 1–3.

Keane, A., Ducette, J., & Adler, D. (1985). Stress in ICU and non-ICU nurses. *Nursing Research, 34*, 231–236.

Killip, T., & Kimball, J. T. (1967). Treatment of myocardial infarction in a coronary care unit: A two-year experience with 250 patients. *American Journal of Cardiology, 20*, 457–464.

Kinney, M. (1981). Survey of critical care nursing practice. Part II. Unit characteristics. *Heart & Lung, 10*, 1051–1054.

Kirchoff, K. J. (1982). Visiting policies for patients with myocardial infarction—a national survey. *Heart & Lung, 11*, 571–576.

Knaus, W. A., Draper, E. A., Wagner, D. P., & Zimmerman, J. E. (1985). APACHE II: A severity of disease classification system. *Critical Care Medicine, 13*, 818–829.

Knaus, W. A., Draper, E. A., Wagner, D. P., Zimmerman, J. E., Birnbaum, M. L., Cullen, D. J., Kohles, M. K., Shin, B., & Snyder, J. V. (1982). Evaluating outcome from intensive care: A preliminary multihospital comparison. *Critical Care Medicine, 10*, 491–496.

Knaus, W. A., LeGall, J. R., Wagner, D. P., Draper, E. A., Loriat, P., Abizanda Campos, R., Cullen, D. J., Kohles, M. K., Glaser, P., Granthil, C., Mercier, P., Nicholas, F., Nikki, P., Shin, B., Snyder, J. V., Wattel, F., & Zimmerman, J. E. (1982). A comparison of intensive care in the U.S.A. and France. *Lancet, 2*, 642–646.

Knaus, W. A., Wagner, D. P., & Draper, E. A. (1985). Relationship between acute physiologic derangement and risk of death. *Journal of Chronic Disease, 4*, 295–300.

Knaus, W. A., Zimmerman, J. E., Wagner, D. P., Draper, E. A., & Lawrence, D. E. (1981). APACHE—acute physiology and chronic health evaluation: A physiologically based classification system. *Critical Care Medicine, 9*, 591–597.

Kornfeld, D. S. (1980). The intensive care unit in adults: Coronary care and general medical/surgical. *Advances in Psychosomatic Medicine, 10*, 1–29.

Kornfeld, D. S., Zimberg, S., & Malm, J. R. (1965). Psychiatric complications of open-heart surgery. *New England Journal of Medicine, 273*, 282–287.

Kotecki, C. I. (1982). Identifying risk of postcardiotomy delirium: A pilot study. *Heart & Lung, 11*, 258–259.

Lasater, K. L., & Grisanti, D. J. (1975). Postcardiotomy psychosis: Indications and interventions. *Heart & Lung, 4*, 724–729.

Layne, O., & Yudofsky, S. (1971). Postoperative psychosis in cardiotomy patients. *New England Journal of Medicine, 284*, 518–520.

LeGall, J. R., Brun-Buisson, C., Trunet, P., Latournerie, J., Chantereau, L., & Rapin, M. (1982). Influence of age, previous health status, and severity of acute illness on outcome from intensive care. *Critical Care Medicine, 10*, 575–577.

LeGall, J. R., Loirat, P., Alperovitch, A., Glaser, P., Granthil, C., Mathieu, D., Mercier, P., Thomas, R., & Villers, D. (1984). A simplified acute physiology score for ICU patients. *Critical Care Medicine, 12*, 975–977.

Leigh, H., Hofer, M. A., & Cooper, J. (1972). A psychological comparison of patients in "open" and "closed" coronary care units. *Journal of Psychosomatic Research, 16*, 449–457.

Lemeshow, S., Teres, D., Pastides, H., Avrunin, J. S., & Steingrub, J. S. (1985). A method for predicting survival and mortality of ICU patients using objectively derived weights. *Critical Care Medicine, 13*, 519–525.

Lester, D., & Brower, E. R. (1981). Stress and job satisfaction in a sample of pediatric intensive care nurses. *Psychological Reports, 48*, 738.

Lewandowski, W., Daly, B., McClish, D. K., Juknialis, B. W., & Youngner, S. J. (1985). Treatment and care of "do not resuscitate" patients in a medical intensive care unit. *Heart & Lung, 14*, 175–186.

Lindquist, R. D., Jeffery, R. W., Johnson, A., & Haus, E. (1985). The stress of patient adjustment to the coronary care unit as related to perceptions of personal control and control preference. *Heart & Lung, 14*, 297–298.

Maloney, J. (1982). Job stress and its consequences on a group of intensive care and nonintensive care nurses. *Advances in Nursing Science, 4*(2), 31–42.

Maloney, J., & Bartz, C. (1983). Stress-tolerant people: Intensive care nurses compared with nonintensive care nurses. *Heart & Lung, 12*, 389-394.

Martino, J. H., & McIntosh, N. J. (1985). Effects of patient characteristics and technology on job satisfaction and stress of intensive care unit and nonintensive care unit nurses. *Heart & Lung, 14*, 300-301.

Mather, H. G., Morgan, D. C., Pearson, N. G., Read, K. L. Q., Shaw, D. B., Steed, G. R., Thorne, M. G., Lawrence, C. J., & Riley, I. S. (1976). Myocardial infarction: A comparison between home and hospital care for patients. *British Medical Journal, 1*, 925-929.

Meffert, H. J., Dahme, B., Flemming, B., Gotze, P., Huse-Kleinstoll, G., Rodewald, G., & Speidel, H. (1980). Open heart surgery from the psychological point of view and resulting therapeutic considerations. *Psychotherapy and Psychosomatics, 32*, 148-156.

Mohl, P. C., Denny, N. R., Mote, T. A., & Coldwater, C. (1982). Hospital unit stressors that affect nurses: Primary task vs. social factors. *Psychosomatics, 23*, 366-374.

Molter, N. C. (1979). Needs of relatives of critically ill patients: A descriptive study. *Heart & Lung, 8*, 332-339.

Montgomery, A. B., Stager, M. A., Carrico, C. J., & Hudson, L. D. (1985). *American Review of Respiratory Disease, 132*, 485-489.

Mulley, A. G., Thibault, G. E., Hughes, R. A., Barnett, G. O., Reder, V. A., & Sherman, E. L. (1980). The course of patients with suspected myocardial infarction: The identification of low risk patients for early transfer from intensive care. *New England Journal of Medicine, 302*, 943-948.

Mulligan, C. D. (1975). Continuing evaluation of coronary care. *Heart & Lung, 4*, 227-232.

Mundt, M. M. (1985). A descriptive study of intensive care unit staff nurses' perceptions of stress in their work environment. *Heart & Lung, 14*, 301-302.

Nastasy, E. L. (1985). Identifying environmental stressors for cardiac surgery patients in a surgical intensive care unit. *Heart & Lung, 14*, 302-303.

Noble, M. A. (1979). Communication in the ICU: Therapeutic or disturbing? *Nursing Outlook, 27*, 195-198.

Norbeck, J. S. (1985). Types and sources of social support for managing job stress in critical care nursing. *Nursing Research, 34*, 225-230.

Norris, R. M., Brandt, P. W. T., Caughey, D. E., Lee, A. J., & Scott, P. J. (1969). A new coronary prognostic index. *Lancet, 1*, 274-278.

Nunn, J. F., Milledge, J. S., & Singaraya, J. (1979). Survival of patients ventilated in an intensive therapy unit. *British Medical Journal, 1*, 1525-1527.

Oskins, S. L. (1979). Identification of situational stressors and coping methods by intensive care nurses. *Heart & Lung, 8*, 953-960.

Parno, J. R., Teres, D., Lemeshow, S., & Brown, R. B. (1982). Hospital charges and long-term survival of ICU versus non-ICU patients. *Critical Care Medicine, 10*, 569-574.

Parno, J. R., Teres, D., Lemeshow, S., Brown, R. B., & Avrunin, J. S. (1984). Two-year outcome of adult intensive care patients. *Medical Care, 22*, 167-176.

Patacky, M. G., Garvin, B. J., & Schwirian, P. M. (1985). Intraaortic balloon pumping and stress in the coronary care unit. *Heart & Lung, 14*, 142-148.

Piper, K. W., & Griner, P. F. (1974). Suicide attempts with drug overdose: Outcomes of intensive vs. conventional floor care. *Archives of Internal Medicine, 134*, 703-706.

Prowse, M. D. (1984). Needs of family members of patients as perceived by family members and nurses in an intensive care unit: An exploratory study. *Heart & Lung, 13*, 310–311.

Redding, J. S., Hargest, T. S., & Minsky, S. H. (1977). How noisy is intensive care? *Critical Care Medicine, 5*, 275–276.

Riggio, R. E., Singer, R. D., Hartman, K., & Sneider, R. (1982). Psychological issues in the care of critically-ill respirator patients: Differential perceptions of patients, relatives, and staff. *Psychological Reports, 51*, 363–369.

Rogers, C. D. (1983). Needs of relatives of cardiac surgery patients during the critical care phase. *Focus on Critical Care, 10*, 50–55.

Rogers, R. M., Weiler, C., & Ruppenthal, B. (1972). Impact of the respiratory intensive care unit on survival of patients with acute respiratory failure. *Chest, 62*, 94–97.

Sadler, P. D. (1979). Nursing assessment of postcardiotomy delirium. *Heart & Lung, 8*, 745–750.

Savage, T., Cullen, D., Kirchhoff, K., & Pugh, B. (1985). Neonatal nurses' responses to "do not resuscitate" orders. *Heart & Lung, 14*, 304–305.

Scheffler, R. M., Knaus, W. A., Wagner, D. P., & Zimmerman, J. E. (1982). Severity of illness and the relationship between intensive care and survival. *American Journal of Public Health, 72*, 449–454.

Schwartz, L. P., & Brenner, Z. R. (1979). Critical care unit transfer: Reducing patient stress through nursing intervention. *Heart & Lung, 8*, 540–546.

Sczekalla, R. M. (1973). Stress reactions of C.C.U. patients to resuscitation procedures on patients. *Nursing Research, 22*, 65–69.

Stange, P. V., & Sumner, A. T. (1978). Predicting treatment costs and life expectancy for end-stage renal disease. *New England Journal of Medicine, 298*, 372–378.

Steffen, S. M. (1980). Perceptions of stress: 1800 nurses tell their stories. In K. E. Claus & J. T. Bailey (Eds.), *Living with stress and promoting well-being* (pp. 38–58). St. Louis: Mosby.

Stehle, J. L. (1981). Critical care nursing stress: The findings revisited. *Nursing Research, 30*, 182–186.

Stillwell, S. B. (1984). Importance of visiting needs of families with relatives in the intensive care unit. *Heart & Lung, 13*, 238–242.

Stone, G. L., Jebsen, P., Walk, P., & Belsham, R. (1984). Identification of stress and coping skills within a critical care setting. *Western Journal of Nursing Research, 6*, 201–211.

Sullivan, S., & Breu, C. (1982). Survey of critical care nursing practice. Part IV. Staffing and training of intensive care unit personnel. *Heart & Lung, 11*, 237–241.

Teres, D., Brown, R. B., & Lemeshow, S. (1982). Predicting mortality of intensive care unit patients: The importance of coma. *Critical Care Medicine, 10*, 86–95.

Thibault, G. E., Mulley, A. G., Barnett, G. O., Goldstein, R. L., Reder, V. A., Sherman, E. L., & Skinner, E. R. (1980). Medical intensive care: Indications, interventions, and outcomes. *New England Journal of Medicine, 302*, 938–492.

Thierer, J., Perhus, S., & McCracken, L. (1981). *Standards for nursing care of the critically ill.* Reston, VA: Reston.

Toth, J. C. (1980). Effect of structured preparation for transfer on patient anxiety. *Nursing Research, 29*, 28-34.

Van der Lelie, J., Endert, E., Wieling, W., & Dunning, A. J. (1981). Is the coronary care unit a coronary scare unit? *Acta Medica Scandinavica, 210*, 497-500.

Vanson, R. J., Katz, B. M., & Krekeler, K. (1980). Stress effects on patients in critical care units from procedures performed on others. *Heart & Lung, 9*, 494-497.

Wagner, D. P., Draper, E. A., Abizanda Campos, R., Nikki, P., LeGall, J. R., Loirat, P., & Knaus, W. A. (1984). Initial international use of APACHE.: An acute severity of disease measure. *Medical Decision Making, 4*, 297-313.

Wagner, D. P., Knaus, W. A., & Draper, E. A. (1983). Statistical validation of a severity of illness measure. *American Journal of Public Health, 73*, 878-884.

Wagner, D. P., Knaus, W. A., & Draper, E. A. (1986). Physiologic abnormalities and outcome from acute disease: Evidence for a predictable relationship. *Archives of Internal Medicine, 146*, 1389-1396.

Warner, J., & Lopez, A. (1985). Factors related to burnout in critical care nurses. *Heart & Lung, 14*, 308.

Whalen, E. R. (1984). Informed consent: The opinions of critical care nurses. *Heart & Lung, 13*, 662-666.

Witek, T. J., Schachter, N., Dean, N. L., & Beck, G. J. (1985). Technically assisted ventilation in a community hospital. *Archives of Internal Medicine, 145*, 235-239.

Witte, K. L. (1984). Variables present in patients who are either resuscitated or not resuscitated in a medical intensive care unit. *Heart & Lung, 13*, 159-163.

PART III

Research on Nursing Education

Chapter 6

Faculty Practice

GRACE H. CHICKADONZ
SCHOOL OF NURSING
MEDICAL COLLEGE OF OHIO

CONTENTS

The involvement of faculty in the practice domain of nursing is a focus of increasing emphasis today. Mauksch (1980, 1981) saw the issue to be of such importance as to label it "a professional imperative." Compelling reasons given for such involvement have been to generate theory, guide clinical research, strengthen teaching, and improve the effectiveness of patient care ("Statement of Belief," 1979). Administrative mechanisms to facilitate faculty involvement in practice have been labeled *unification models*. Such models referred to the collaborative efforts of nurse administrators and educators to advance nursing as a practice discipline in the three areas of practice, teaching, and research.

The development of unification models has been in process in several institutions for many years. As early as 1959 Smith (1959,

1965, 1985) described the seeds of faculty practice and the first unification effort at the University of Florida. Similar efforts followed. Schlotfeldt and MacPhail (1969a, 1969b, 1969c) introduced an "experiment in nursing" at Case Western Reserve University emphasizing academic leadership and planned change as the process for achieving integration of practice, education, and research; the development of that project has been described in subsequent writings (Fitzpatrick, 1985; Fitzpatrick & Halloran, 1985; Fitzpatrick, Halloran, & Algase, in press; MacPhail, 1975, 1980, 1981; Pierik, 1971, 1973; Schlotfeldt, 1981). Ford and her colleagues at the University of Rochester described the use of a unification model in developing a center of excellence for integrating nursing practice, education, and research (Ford, 1980, 1981a, 1981b, 1981c, 1985; Ford & Kitzman, 1983; Sovie, 1981a, 1981b). In developing the unification effort at Rush University Christman (1979, 1980, 1985) addressed the need for professional models of practice. More recently, at Rutgers University, Joel (1985) described a contractual agreement approach and emphasized the importance of each institution creating its own effort rather than attempting to duplicate models designed by other institutions. Finally, Fagin (1985) described the University of Pennsylvania partnership plan, which differentiates the roles of clinician–educator faculty and investigator–educator faculty.

Action to move faculty practice forward within the profession has been enhanced significantly through programs to prepare nurse faculty for practice roles and to provide opportunity to develop professional networks and share scholarly work. The Robert Wood Johnson (RWJ) Nurse Faculty Fellowship in Primary Care Program (Keenan, 1985; Mauksch, 1985; Williams & Lindeman, 1985) and, subsequently, the RWJ Clinical Scholars Program were designed to prepare nursing faculty for clinical practice and research in primary care and hospital settings. The Annual Symposium on Faculty Practice, established by the American Academy of Nursing (Barnard, 1983; Barnard & Smith, 1985) was designed to give visibility to the importance of faculty practice and to provide for the exchange of ideas. These endeavors brought together faculty who were interested in the practice of nursing as an inherent part of the faculty role and created a forum for exploring the related issues. The increasing attention to faculty practice and unification models over a period of 20 years seemed to warrant a critical review of research on the topic.

The identification of published research was begun through a computerized search of the nursing literature, using the key words *faculty practice* and *unification*. Twenty-eight relevant articles were identified; the references cited in each were evaluated, and an additional forty-eight articles were located. Authors of unpublished works were contacted to ascertain if papers had been published. Only six published research papers were identified from the literature search, indicating the enormous gap between a changing role of major importance and the availability of answers through research to guide the change. The six published studies are reviewed in three sections on types of faculty practice, factors affecting faculty practice, and receptivity to faculty practice and the unification of nursing education and service.

TYPES OF FACULTY PRACTICE

The characteristics of faculty group practices were studied by Rosswurm (1981). Twenty-three faculty practices were identified through deans of schools of nursing that offered nurse practitioner programs. A nurse–faculty group practice was defined as one in which "a faculty group works as a team to deliver direct care to clients" (p. 327). Data were sought about characteristics of the practice, the nurses in the practice, the clients served, and the major benefits and problems experienced.

The major benefits cited by the nurses in the practice were independence, enjoyment and excitement of practicing nursing, maintaining clinical skills, and role model for students. The major problems identified were scheduling problems for teaching and practice and lack of third party reimbursement. Most of the practices were not based on a particular theoretical model; however, 7 of the 23 practices were based on Orem's model (1985), and the most research was in process in those practices. Some faculty appeared to be incorporating activities of teaching, research, and practice into a single role.

Weaknesses of the study were related to the limited number of schools surveyed, inclusion of only those with nurse practitioner programs, and lack of clearly defined terms to describe the practices. Also missing were in-depth data about the practices, such as the number of clients seen, the financial base, the types of services provided, the outcomes of care, the satisfaction of consumers and nurse faculty, and the presence of teaching and research activities.

A second type of faculty practice, the joint appointment, was addressed by Davis and Tomney (1982). A joint appointment was defined as "one agreed to by two or more institutions where the appointee holds a position in each institution and carries out a defined responsibility in each" (p. 34). Results from a questionnaire to deans of schools of nursing in Canada revealed that 10 of the 16 schools in Canada had jointly appointed positions of two types: cost-shared and non-cost-shared. Acute care hospitals were the partners most commonly identified with the school in the joint appointment. The study had serious limitations in the definition of terms, the characteristics of the joint appointments, and the lack of in-depth data about the roles described.

The description of faculty group practices and the identification of joint appointments in Canadian university nursing programs are interesting first steps in research about faculty practice. Further research is needed to describe joint appointment practices within the United States as well as to describe other models of nursing practice, for instance, institutional collaboration and independent practice.

FACTORS AFFECTING FACULTY PRACTICE

The problems of faculty practice and factors inhibiting or facilitating faculty practice were addressed in two 1983 studies (Anderson & Pierson; Dickens). Anderson and Pierson based their research on role theory and addressed the need of students to see the faculty member as a role model who was both knowledgeable in an area of nursing practice and capable of demonstrating clinical skills. This study provided the most comphrensive descriptive data to date on faculty practice, and, consequently, is reviewed in detail. Faculty who practiced were identified through a query letter to deans of 127 National League for Nursing-accredited baccalaureate programs. Completed questionnaires were returned by 573 of the 972 faculty comprising the final sample. Faculty practice was defined as "clinical practice involving a faculty member with the health care of clients. . . . This practice should be over and above the expected clinical teaching role" (p. 132).

The additional term of *moonlighting* was used to designate "clinical practice not contracted by or through the school of nursing" (p. 132).

Results of the study indicated that 18% of the respondents practiced only during summer and vacation periods. Over half of the remaining subjects averaged 8 hours or less per week in practice, and the majority were not engaged in research or professional writing. The median weekly workload was 45.6 hours. The findings indicated that enriching teaching, maintaining clinical skills, and personal satisfaction were the most important reasons to practice. Of least importance were reasons related to research or curriculum. Economic reasons were not offered as choices. Seventeen percent of the sample indicated that they held joint appointments; 48% used moonlighting as the way of accomplishing faculty practice. Hospitals were the most frequently used setting (58%). Thirty-seven percent of respondents reported that the school philosophy included faculty practice, but 58% of the total sample indicated that no time was allocated for practice. Only 19% of the sample reported that the school had authority and accountability over the setting in which faculty were engaged in practice. Among schools attached to a health science center, the figure increased to 29%.

Fifty-five faculty (10% of the respondents) reported that there was a reimbursement policy for faculty practice, but only 32 of these respondents indicated that the policy allowed for an additional source of income to the faculty member from the practice. Twenty-six percent indicated that there were criteria for evaluating the practice component.

Salary supplementation was viewed by the respondents as a facilitator of practice. Administrators were viewed as the greatest facilitator and workload as the primary inhibitor. Almost all of the respondents reported that students responded positively to the faculty's practice. However, half indicated that faculty colleages responded negatively.

In comparing the responses of faculty from two schools where a unification model was used ($n = 71$) with those from schools where other models were used ($n = 501$), there was no difference in terms of total hours of weekly workload. However, administrators were seen as facilitators of faculty practice by a higher proportion of unification model (UM) faculty than other faculty and as inhibitors of practice by a higher proportion of other faculty than UM faculty. The reactions of service personnel to faculty practice also were judged differently, with service personnel seen as less supportive by UM faculty than by other faculty.

The authors recommended future research in several areas: attitudes of hospital administrators and service personnel, satisfaction of faculty with specific models, factors affecting workload, impact on clients and students, and the perceptions of nonpracticing faculty toward maintaining clinical skills. The need for pretest–posttest designs for research on schools developing unification models was cited also.

Anderson and Pierson's (1983) study was limited by the lack of development of the role theory concept, lack of clarity in terminology, and the sample selection procedures. The omission of data regarding summer employment, economic benefits of faculty practice, and research and scholarly activity were also limitations. The striking and most disturbing finding lay in the reasons given by respondents for faculty practice. If impact on curricula and clinical nursing research were not important reasons for faculty practice, one could question seriously the value of the effort expended by both administrators and faculty to achieve faculty practice. Equally disturbing was the moonlighting of 48% of the practicing faculty, indicating that the school was not involved officially in facilitating practice opportunities for faculty.

Dickens (1983) acknowledged the ambivalence of faculty about becoming involved in practice and examined existing mechanisms of social support for faculty who practiced. The study was based on the views of Chickadonz, Bush, Korthius, and Utz (1981), who outlined the changes needed to incorporate practice into faculty roles, and on House's (1981) operationalization of supportive behaviors: informational, emotional, instrumental, and appraisal support (Dickens, 1983).

A survey was conducted of nursing administrators for schools with baccalaureate and master's degree programs in the southeastern United States, with responses from 74 of the 113 administrators in the sample. Administrators reported that 32% of their full-time faculty and 42% of their part-time faculty were involved in clinical practice in the 1981–1982 academic year. The types of clinical practice in which the faculty were involved included joint appointments, private practice, group practice, nursing clinics, and others. The largest number of full-time faculty (52%) were involved in "other" practices, identified as summer, weekend, and recess practice in various health agencies. The largest number of part-time faculty (46%) were involved in joint appointments.

Conclusions drawn from the data indicated that there was limited evidence of instrumental, informational, or appraisal support for faculty who practiced. Some evidence of emotional support was identified. Although the study was limited in design, sample, and development of the conceptual framework, Dickens probed one step further by exploring the existence of forms of social support for faculty who practiced. It was interesting to note again that over half of the 32% of the faculty who were practicing were doing so in summer, recess, or on weekends.

It is clear that both more support and more research are needed if schools are to be successful in achieving faculty practice. In each of the studies cited thus far, a question is raised about what activities should constitute faculty practice. Clear definitions of terms are essential if study findings are to be meaningful.

RECEPTIVITY TO A UNIFICATION MODEL
FOR FACULTY PRACTICE

It was evident from the studies described thus far that, although faculty practice and unification models do exist, they neither have been adopted widely nor studied. The last two papers originated from one project to address the question of receptivity to a unification model for practice among nursing faculty in the United States (Yarcheski & Mahon, 1985, 1986). According to Yarcheski and Mahon, in the status-risk theory receptivity to change has been proposed as a function of status or position held and the degree to which an innovation either threatens or benefits the person's status. The degree of receptivity was examined first among groups of deans, tenured faculty, and nontenured faculty (1985); subsequently, receptivity was examined within each group (1986).

A systematic random sampling procedure was used to identify 298 educators drawn from baccalaureate nursing programs accredited by the National League for Nursing for 1982–1983. Two hundred and twenty-two (75%) returned usable responses, including 72 deans, 64 tenured faculty, and 86 nontenured faculty.

A description of a unification model was developed that included the purposes, organizational arrangements, dean and faculty responsibilities, and arrangements for workloads and practice activities. Participants were asked to respond to the description by completing three semantic differential instruments as if the unification model were to be adopted in their setting. Results of the study did not indicate significant differences among deans, tenured faculty, and nontenured faculty. However, the means obtained on receptivity to the model indicated that greater receptivity existed among nontenured faculty, followed by the deans and then tenured faculty. There were high correlations between receptivity to unification and both the level of direct risk or benefit perceived and the level of indirect risk or benefit perceived.

Yarcheski and Mahon's study was the first systematic attempt to assess receptivity to unification. The use of the status-risk theory of receptivity was useful in forming a framework for the study. The major limitation of the study was the inadequacy of the theory and the literature in providing direct descriptions of risks and benefits perceived by the three groups. The generation of hypotheses without such a base left the researchers in the position of operating only from logic.

In the second study, Yarcheski and Mahon (1986) used the same data base to analyze receptivity within the groups of deans, tenured faculty, and nontenured faculty. In addition, they examined selected nonorganizational and informal organizational statuses in an attempt to explain receptivity to the proposed introduction of the unification model. The informal organizational status variables examined included basic nursing education, present educational preparation, and whether one's academic institution required a doctorate for tenure. The nonorganizational status variables examined were marital status, parental status, and age.

From the statistically significant results related to receptivity and status variables, the authors summarized their findings as follows: (a) In the group of deans, no informal organizational or nonorganizational status variables were identified as risk–receptivity factors; parental status was related positively at a low level to receptivity to unification. (b) Tenured faculty whose academic affiliation required a doctorate projected significantly less receptivity to the unification model and significantly less effective performance in the combined roles than those tenured faculty whose academic affiliation did not require a doctorate. The number of years of experience in nursing service and age were related inversely at a low level to receptivity and performance. (c) Among nontenured faculty, faculty who were doctorally prepared were significantly less receptive to the unification model than those who were master's prepared and also rated themselves lower on effectiveness in combining roles. Also, nontenured faculty whose academic institution required a doctorate for tenure perceived significantly greater risk than those whose institutions did not require a doctorate. Their risk perceptions, however, did not change their receptivity to the model. Finally, weak to moderate inverse relationships were found between the number of years of experience in nursing education and both receptivity and risk. The strength of this study was the identification of variables within the groups of tenured and nontenured faculty that accounted for different levels of receptivity and perceived risk to introduction of the unification model.

SUMMARY AND PROJECTIONS

The six studies reviewed constitute all of the published research on faculty practice and unification models. The studies are descriptive research that only begin to address the questions related to faculty practice and unification models. The results indicate that some faculty practice is occurring and that there are varying degrees of receptivity to introducing the unification model. The need for future research is striking. One problem in developing a paradigm for future work is the lack of theoretical conceptualizations for much of the existing writing and research. Fagin (1985, p. 14) describes the most comprehensive framework: "As we look to the future, any new organizational design for institutionalizing practice must be accompanied by a plan for research as to outcome in the stated goals . . . education, research, nursing practice, and professionalism." In addition to acknowledging agreement with Fagin's four areas, Ford (1985) suggests that models, and thus frameworks for research, also may be derived from values, functions, and philosophy, as well as from structural or organizational theory. Five areas for future research are discussed below: the expansion of faculty practice, case studies of unification models, impact studies, social context studies, and studies on faculty who practice.

Expansion of Faculty Practice

Surveys are needed to describe accurately the extent to which faculty practice and unification models are being developed within schools of nursing. Clear definition of terms is essential for such data to be meaningful. For example, working summers and weekends for additional compensation or to maintain clinical skills has been one operational definition of faculty practice. However, that perspective is entirely different from the perspective of faculty engaged in practice who are in control of their practice sites, have students involved in learning experiences with them, produce clinical research about their work, and are compensated for their services. Interpretation of data collected from these two diverse perspectives must include consideration of the differences. Variables to be taken into account include geographic region, types of schools (public, private; health science centers, liberal arts colleges; undergraduate and graduate programs), faculty demographic data (numbers of faculty; characteristics of faculty involved, such as personal data and educational levels), and types of models (collaboration, unification, faculty practice). Other variables included should address the types of practice sites, clients served, economic base for the practice, and activities related to teaching, theory generation, and research.

Just as this chapter was being completed, data of this type were published by the Generic Baccalaureate Nursing Data Project sponsored by the American Association of Colleges of Nursing (Redman, Cassells, & Jackson, 1985). In a 1984 questionnaire, deans were asked to describe practice related to the faculty role. Results reported in three areas are relevant to this chapter. Seventy-nine of 246 deans indicated that faculty are provided time during the work week for clinical practice. Areas of collaboration between nursing faculty and clinical agencies and the perceived benefits of that collaboration also were identified. Some faculty held joint or shared appointments in 68 of the participating schools, and the positions generate revenue for 15 schools. This type of survey data is needed to monitor the evolution of faculty practice in university schools of nursing.

Case Studies of Unification Models

Despite the fairly extensive literature about faculty practice and unification, there has been no comprehensive framework devised and used to review the existing models. Such a framework would need to encompass process, organizational structure, and outcome components in relation to teaching, practice, and research. The existing literature is perhaps sufficient to provide a baseline from which to construct a framework. Case studies of existing and evolving models of faculty practice would be an important contribution. Variables to be addressed might include the following: (a) process — goals, strategies for organizational change, timetables, leadership characteristics, problems, and incentives; (b) structure — characteristics of the models, changes in organizational structure and roles, financing, and descriptions of the practice areas; and (c) outcome — impact on school, faculty, curricula, students, patients, delivery systems, and research.

Impact Studies

The reasons most frequently given for why faculty should practice relate to theory generation, clinical research, strengthening of teaching, and improved patient care. Research is needed to explore whether these outcomes are achieved if faculty do practice, and to guide the development of practice models so that desired outcomes are achieved. Inherent in such studies must be descriptions of the actual practice activities of faculty such as services provided, types of clients served, and reimbursement mechanisms. For example, Kogan, Betrus, Wolf-Wilets, and Elmore (1985) describe a nursing practice center at the University of Washington that fulfills the purpose of practice, teaching, and research.

Another aspect to be examined is the economic impact of faculty practice. This should include benefits to the individual faculty member, impact on the school and nursing service budgets, and benefits to the education and service institutions. In addition, the actual impact of faculty practice on patient care also must be understood. The impact on students, their learning, and their assumption of role behaviors emanating from role modeling is critical.

Monitoring the impact of faculty practice on the development of clinical nursing research is an important area for study. Research productivity and other scholarship can be measured quantitatively by the amount of research and funding for research and through the number and quality of publications. Monitoring the impact of faculty practice on clinical issues in the discipline and the design of research to address these issues in order to structure the body of knowledge is more difficult.

Social Context Studies

Changes in health care today provide a context in which to address the need for faculty practice. Changing reimbursement and delivery systems and patterns of access to care, increasing acuity of illness in patients in institutional and community care, and diminishing resources for health care raise many social issues. Why faculty must practice in this changing milieu is essential to explore. The impact of faculty practice and unification on the image of nursing in the public domain should be monitored closely. The potential is great for improving the image of nursing by having nurse faculty who provide leadership in addressing health care concerns in society and demonstrate to the public the contributions of nursing practice to patient care, teaching, and research.

Faculty Who Practice

More understanding is needed about the characteristics of faculty who choose to practice: their philosophies, values, motivations and rewards, levels of clinical competence, educational preparation and credentials, and factors that facilitate and inhibit their practice. A clearer understanding of the risks and benefits of practice perceived by faculty is essential for creating planned organizational change to accomplish faculty practice and the unification of nursing education and service.

This chapter has provided an overview of faculty practice-related research done to date, including the studies about unification models for faculty practice. Much research is needed to guide the change as an increasing number of schools of nursing address the issues inherent in faculty practice. Suggestions for future research have been presented.

REFERENCES

Anderson, E. R., & Pierson, P. (1983). An exploratory study of faculty practice: Views of those faculty engaged in practice who teach in an NLN accredited baccalaureate program. *Western Journal of Nursing Research, 5*, 129–143.

Barnard, K. E. (Ed.). (1983). *Structure to outcome: Making it work.* Kansas City, MO: American Academy of Nursing.

Barnard, K. E., & Smith, G. R. (Eds.). (1985). *Faculty practice in action*. Kansas City, MO: American Academy of Nursing.

Chicadonz, G. H., Bush, E. E., Korthius, K., & Utz, S. (1981). Mobilizing faculty toward integration of practice into faculty roles. *Nursing Health Care, 2*, 548–553.

Christman, L. (1979). The practitioner–teacher. *Nurse Educator, 4*(2), 8–11.

Christman, L. (1980). Leadership in practice. *Image, 12*, 31–33.

Christman, L. (1985). Response to "Institutionalizing practice: Historical and future perspectives." In K. E. Barnard & G. R. Smith (Eds.), *Faculty practice in action*, (pp. 24–28). Kansas City, MO: American Academy of Nursing.

Davis, L., & Tomney, P. (1982). The best of two worlds. *The Canadian Nurse, 78*, 34–37.

Dickens, M. R. (1983). Faculty practice and social support. *Nursing Leadership, 6*, 121–127.

Fagin, C. (1985). Institutionalizing practice: Historical and future perspectives. In K. E. Barnard & G. R. Smith (Eds.), *Faculty practice in action*, (pp. 1–17). Kansas City, MO: American Academy of Nursing.

Fitzpatrick, J. J. (1985). Response to "Institutionalizing practice: Historical and future perspectives." *Faculty practice in action* (pp. 28–30). Kansas City, MO: American Academy of Nursing.

Fitzpatrick, J. J., & Halloran, E. J. (1985). Proactivating a collaborative service education climate. In *MAIN Proceedings Thriving or Surviving? Managing Pro-Active Environments for Nursing* (pp. 29–41). Indianapolis: Midwest Alliance in Nursing.

Fitzpatrick, J. J., Halloran, E. J., & Algase, D. L. (in press). An experiment in nursing revisited. *Nursing Outlook*.

Ford, L. C. (1980). Unification of nursing practice, education and research. *International Nursing Review, 27*, 178–192.

Ford, L. C. (1981a). Closing the gap between service and education. In I. G. Mauksch (Ed.), *Primary care: A contemporary nursing perspective* (pp. 31–40). New York: Grune & Stratton.

Ford, L. C. (1981b). On the scene: University of Rochester Medical Center. *Nursing Administration Quarterly, 5*, 1–51.

Ford, L. C. (1981c). Creating a center of excellence in nursing. In L. H. Aiken (Ed.), *Health policy and nursing practice* (pp. 242–255). New York: McGraw-Hill.

Ford, L. C. (1985). Response to "Institutionalizing practice: Historical and future perspectives." In K. E. Barnard & G. R. Smith (Eds.), *Faculty practice in action* (pp. 17–23). Kansas City, MO: American Academy of Nursing.

Ford, L. C., & Kitzman, H. J. (1983). Organizational perspectives on faculty practice: Issues and challenges. In K. E. Barnard (Ed.), *Structure to outcome: Making it work* (pp. 13–30). Kansas City, MO: American Academy of Nursing.

House, J. S. (1981). *Work stress and social support*. Reading, MA: Addison-Wesley.

Joel, L. (1985). The Rutgers experience: One perspective on service-education collaboration. *Nursing Outlook, 33*, 220–224.

Keenan, T. (1985). Experiment in role restructuring toward practice: Introduction. In K. E. Barnard & G. R. Smith (Eds.), *Faculty practice in action* (pp. 139–140). Kansas City, MO: American Academy of Nursing.

Kogan, H. N., Betrus, P., Wolf-Wilets, V., & Elmore, S. (1985). Nurse practice centers: Ingredients of success. In K. E. Barnard & G. R. Smith (Eds.), *Faculty practice in action* (pp. 229–245). Kansas City, MO: American Academy of Nursing.

MacPhail, J. (1975). Promoting collaboration between education/service. *The Canadian Nurse, 71*, 32–34.

MacPhail, J. (1980). Promoting collaboration/unification models for nursing education and service. *Cognitive dissonance: Interpreting and implementing faculty practice roles in nursing education* (pp. 33–36). New York: National League for Nursing.

MacPhail, J. (1981). Implementation and evaluation of the Case Western Reserve University unification model. In L. H. Aiken (Ed.), *Health policy and nursing practice* (pp. 229–241). New York: McGraw-Hill.

Mauksch, I. (1980). Faculty practice: A professional imperative. *Nurse Educator, 5*, 21–24.

Mauksch, I. (1981). A rationale for the reunification of nursing services and nursing education. In L. H. Aiken (Ed.), *Health policy and nursing practice* (pp. 211–217). New York: McGraw-Hill.

Mauksch, I. (1985). Experiment in role restructuring toward practice: The Robert Wood Johnson Nurse Faculty Fellowships Program Revisited. In K. E. Barnard & G. R. Smith (Eds.), *Faculty practice in action* (pp. 141–146). Kansas City, MO: American Academy of Nursing.

Orem, D. E. (1985). *Nursing Concepts of Practice*. New York: McGraw-Hill.

Pierik, M. M. (1971). Experiment to effect change. *Supervisor Nurse, 2*, 69–75.

Pierik, M. M. (1973). Joint appointments: Collaboration for better patient care. *Nursing Outlook, 21*, 576–579.

Redman, B. K., Cassells, J. M., & Jackson, S. S. (1985). Generic baccalaureate nursing programs: Survey of enrollment, administrative structure/funding, faculty teaching/practice roles, and selected curriculum trends. *Journal of Professional Nursing, 1*, 369–380.

Rosswurm, M. A. (1981). Characteristics of 23 faculty group nurse practices. *Nursing and Health Care, 2*, 327–330.

Schlotfeldt, R. M. (1981). The development of a model for unifying nursing practice and nursing education. In L. H. Aiken (Ed.), *Health policy and nursing practice* (pp. 218–228). New York: McGraw-Hill.

Schlotfeldt, R. M., & MacPhail, J. (1969a). An experiment in nursing: Rationale and characteristics. *American Journal of Nursing, 69*, 1018–1023.

Schlotfeldt, R. M., & MacPhail, J. (1969b). An experiment in nursing: Introducing planned change. *American Journal of Nursing, 69*, 1247–1251.

Schlotfeldt, R. M., & MacPhail, J. (1969c). An experiment in nursing: Implementing planned change. *American Journal of Nursing, 69*, 1475–1480.

Smith, D. M. (1959). Practice—a part of teaching. *Nursing Outlook, 7*(3), 134–135.

Smith, D. M. (1965). Education and service under one administration. *Nursing Outlook, 13*(2), 54–56.

Smith, D. M. (1985). Response: Faculty practice from a 25-year perspective. In K. E. Barnard & G. R. Smith (Eds.), *Faculty practice in action* (pp. 30–32). Kansas City, MO: American Academy of Nursing.

Sovie, M. D. (1981a). Unifying education and practice: One medical center's design. Part 1. *Journal of Nursing Administration, 11*(1), 41–49.

Sovie, M. D. (1981b). Unifying education and practice: One medical center's design. Part 2. *Journal of Nursing Administration, 11*(2), 30–32.

Statement of Belief Regarding Faculty Practice. (1979). *Nursing Outlook, 27*, 158.

Williams, C. A., & Lindeman, C. A. (1985). Experiment in role restructuring toward practice: Evaluation of the fellowship experience and its impact on roles. In K. E. Barnard & G. R. Smith (Eds.), *Faculty practice in action* (pp. 146–158). Kansas City, MO: American Academy of Nursing.

Yarcheski, A., & Mahon, N. E. (1985). The unification model in nursing: A study of receptivity among nurse educators in the United States. *Nursing Research, 34*, 120–125.

Yarcheski, A., & Mahon, N. E. (1986). The unification model in nursing: Risk-receptivity profiles among deans, tenured and nontenured faculty in the United States. *Western Journal of Nursing Research, 8*, 63–81.

Chapter 7

Teaching Clinical Judgment

CHRISTINE A. TANNER
SCHOOL OF NURSING
OREGON HEALTH SCIENCES UNIVERSITY

CONTENTS

Nurse educators have assigned substantial importance to the teaching of clinical judgment. Objectives for student learning in relation to components of the nursing process are set forth in virtually every undergraduate nursing curriculum (Santora, 1980). National League for Nursing *Criteria for the Evaluation of Baccalaureate and Higher Degree Programs in Nursing (1983)* include specific criteria for incorporating clinical decision making and the nursing process into the undergraduate curriculum. In a recent Delphi survey of research priorities in nursing education, strategies for teaching clinical problem solving were identified as the second highest priority topic of 63 listed

The author gratefully acknowledges the assistance of the following individuals: Karen Padrick, Donnajo Putzier, and Una E. Westfall, co-investigators on the research project "Diagnostic Reasoning in Nursing: An Analysis of Cognitive Strategies," who contributed in many ways to the ideas in this chapter; Ivo Abraham, Doris Carnevali, Sheila Corcoran, and William Holzemer, who provided valuable suggestions on earlier versions of this chapter.

(Tanner & Lindeman, in press). The purpose of this review is to summarize and evaluate nursing research related to the teaching of clinical judgment and to propose directions for future research.

For the purpose of this review, the definition of clinical judgment was adapted from the work of Kelly (1966) as a series of decisions made by the nurse in interaction with the client, regarding (a) the type of observations to be made in the client situation, (b) the evaluation of the data observed and derivation of meaning (diagnosis), and (c) nursing actions that should be taken with or on behalf of the client (management). Subsumed under the rubric of clinical judgment were the frequently used terms of clinical problem solving, clinical decision making, and nursing process.

To be selected for this review, a study was required to meet four criteria. First, the major purpose of the study was deemed relevant to the topic of teaching clinical judgment. Included were studies designed to describe what the processes of clinical judgment are, and, therefore, presumably what processes should be taught; to develop and test measures of clinical judgment performance; to evaluate specific teaching methods; or to identify factors associated with performance. Second, empirical evidence related to the major research questions was provided in the report. Third, subjects were either nursing students or practicing nurses. And fourth, subject performance was described or measured on one or more components of clinical judgment, defined as observation, diagnosis, or management.

Only research published or accepted for publication between 1966 and 1986 was included. The year 1966 was selected because in that year the first major and most frequently cited series of theoretical papers and studies on clinical judgment in nursing was published (Hammond, Kelly, Castellan, Schneider, & Vancini, 1966; Hammond, Kelly, Schneider, & Vancini, 1966a, 1966b, 1967; Kelly, 1966). Literature retrieval strategies included computer searches of MEDLINE and PsychINFO, manual searches of nursing indexes, issue-by-issue review of journals that publish nursing research, examination of the proceedings of the National Conferences on Classification of Research on Nursing Diagnoses (Gebbie & Lavin, 1975; Kim, McFarland, & McLane, 1984; Kim & Moritz, 1982), review of the reference lists in retrieved literature, and informal contacts made by the author.

The 53 published studies that met the inclusion criteria were categorized into four groupings according to the major purpose of the study. Nineteen (36%) of the publications were focused on describing the processes of clinical judgment. Twelve (23%) were reports of methodological research, testing five measures of clinical judgment performance. The effectiveness of teaching methods in improving student or nurse performance in clinical judgment was evaluated in only five (9%) of the studies. The final category included the 17 reports (32%) in which the major emphasis was the identification of factors associated with clinical judgment performance.

Each of the studies was evaluated for scientific merit using the following general criteria: clarity of study questions and underlying conceptualization; appropriateness of study methods; including design, sample, instruments, and analytic procedures for the study question and conceptualization; and clarity and logic of the interpretation and conclusions. Studies are included in the review even if some of these criteria are not met; specific methodological and conceptual issues are identified for studies in which they seriously jeopardized the validity of the results. Following the review and evaluation of the research in each of the four categories, all studies are analyzed for commonalities in methodological issues, underlying assumptions, and their overall contribution to the knowledge base for the teaching of clinical judgment. The review is concluded with suggested directions for future research.

PROCESSES OF CLINICAL JUDGMENT

Many investigators have argued cogently that an understanding of the processes of clinical judgment is a necessary prerequisite to the development of suitable instructional methods for teaching those processes (Broderick & Ammentorp, 1979; Corcoran, 1986a; Gordon, 1980; Hammond et al., 1967; Pyles & Stern, 1983; Westfall, Tanner, Putzier, & Padrick, 1986). Two aspects of the processes of clinical judgment seem particularly useful as a basis for instructional decisions: (a) an understanding of how competent individuals proceed in determining what observations to make, in identifying health problems from those observations, and in deciding on appropriate actions; and (b) an understanding of the progression of such competence, from beginning level to the development of expertise.

Although many studies on the processes of clinical judgment were reviewed within the context of information processing for nursing practice in a prior volume of the *Annual Review of Nursing Research* (Grier, 1984), they are included in this review for two purposes: (a) to determine the extent to which descriptive theories of clinical judgment have been tested adequately in nursing to provide guidance for instructional innovation; and (b) to examine shared findings from theoretically divergent studies, specifically in the area of the development of expertise in clinical judgment.

Descriptive Theories

Hammond and his associates conducted the first major series of studies on the process of clinical inference in nursing (Hammond, 1966; Hammond, Kelly, Castellan, Schneider, & Vancini, 1966; Hammond, Kelly, Schneider, & Vancini, 1966a, 1966b, 1967). Hammond (1966) defined clinical inference as the process of identifying the unobservable "state of the patient" from unobservable data. The task of clinical inference was described as complex to the extent that the data have an uncertain, probabilistic relationship to the patient state. Hammond and associates expected to detect patterns among nurses in their use of cues for identifying patient states. They also expected that these patterns would vary as a function of task complexity. However, in two studies (Hammond, Kelly, Schneider, & Vancini, 1966a, 1966b) the selection of actions by nurses was not related to the recognition of any single cue or to groupings of cues. In short, no pattern of inference could be found.

Hammond and associates introduced two theoretical perspectives to the study of clinical judgment in nursing, concept attainment theory and statistical decision theory (Hammond, Kelly, Castellan, Schneider, & Vancini, 1966; Hammond et al., 1967). Each of these theories has been used as the basis for a limited number of additional studies in nursing.

Concept attainment theory has its origins in the work of Bruner, Goodnow, and Austin (1956). The theory describes cognitive strategies that humans use to form categories or concepts when confronted with a set of descriptors. Humans attend selectively to information, formulate hypotheses about possible ways to categorize the information, and select a strategy to test the hypotheses. According to the theory, the strategy selected, in part, is a function of the amount and relevance of information available. In three studies, (Cianfrani, 1984; Gordon, 1980; Matthews & Gaul, 1979) investigators used this theory as a "framework," although none clearly identified their study as a test of the theory or of its applicability to clinical judgment.

Gordon (1980) found that nurse subjects used hypothesis-testing strategies similar to those described in the concept attainment literature on a diagnostic test. However, the selection of strategies did not vary as a function of information conditions as predicted by the theory. Cianfrani (1984), however, found that the number of health problems identified and the accuracy of diagnosis did vary as a function of the amount and relevance of the information. In a somewhat different approach, Matthews and Gaul (1979) examined the usefulness of the concept attainment perspective by testing the relationship between overall concept attainment ability and cue perception in a nursing diagnosis task. There was a positive relationship between scores on a concept mastery test and diagnostic scores on a case study for undergraduate student subjects, but not for graduate students. Whether the process of diagnosis in general and, specifically, hypothesis testing and information gathering can be described adequately using the concept attainment model has not been resolved by these three studies.

Two statistical models of decision making, Bayes' theorem and utility theory, have been used extensively in studies of physicians in two ways: descriptively, to compare clinicians' decisions with those derived by the model, and normatively, to prescribe appropriate decisions. Each of the models has been used in a single study of nurses' performance. Bayes' theorem described a way in which judgments could be revised optimally in light of new information. Hammond et al. (1967) found that nurses tended to revise probabilities in the direction suggested by the theorem, but the amount of revision was much less than that prescribed by the model. Utility theory described the selection of actions based on subjective assignments of value to certain outcomes and of the probability of the occurrence of those outcomes given certain actions. Using this theory, Grier (1976) found that nurses' intuitive judgments agreed with the actions prescribed by the model in the majority of cases.

A third theoretical framework used in the study of clinical judgment is that of information processing theory. In this theory problem solving is described as an interaction between an information processing system, the problem solver, a task environment, and the task as described by the experimenter (Newell & Simon, 1972). The major assumption underlying the theory is that there are limits to human information processing capacity; effective problem solving rests on the individual's ability to adapt to these limitations. In three studies, investigators have attempted to describe the strategies nursing students or nurses use to adapt their limited resources to the demands of a complex task environment. The strategy of activating diagnostic hypotheses as a means to narrow the range of information needed, and hence to reduce task complexity, is described in two studies of nursing students (Tanner, 1982; Westfall et al., 1986) and one of practicing nurses (Westfall et al., 1986). Corcoran (1986a, 1986b) has described the use of an "opportunistic," as opposed to a systematic, approach to planning nursing care; presumably the opportunistic strategy, which is used by experts in more complex tasks, conserves limited information-processing resources.

In addition to studies related to these major theoretical perspectives, inductive approaches also have been applied to the study of clinical judgment in nursing (Baumann & Bourbonnais, 1982; Benner, 1984; Benner & Wrubel, 1982; Phillips & Rempusheski, 1985; Pyles & Stern, 1983). Benner (1984) described seven domains of skilled performance in nursing; among those which were directly related to clinical judgment in nursing were the helping role, the teaching–coaching function, the diagnostic and patient–monitoring function, and effective management of rapidly changing situations. Of particular interest to this review was what Benner and Wrubel (1982) described as a "grasp of the whole situation," a qualitative or perceptual assessment based on a combination of input from the senses and interpretation of the patient's physical, verbal, and behavioral expressions. This description was similar to what Pyles and Stern (1983) identified as the formation of a "gestalt" or the achievement of insight about a patient situation. Both groups of investigators identified the intuitive grasp or formation of a gestalt as characteristic of expert performance.

It is clear that a wide range of theoretical perspectives has been used as the basis for relatively few studies. Virtually all investigators have claimed in their conclusions empirical support for the theory tested, although most recognize that additional study is needed. In 20 years of research, no single theory has been investigated sufficiently to conclude that the theory can be supported or refuted, or that it is in need of revision. Hence, the goal of describing the processes of clinical judgment as a prerequisite to instructional design has not yet been achieved.

Development of Expertise

A relatively recent focus of inquiry that is shared by investigators using both information processing theory and inductive approaches is the comparison of performance between novice and experts. Such comparisons may prove useful both theoretically, in understanding how expertise develops, and practically, in the design of instructional methods for differing levels of students and clinicians.

In studies of diagnostic inferences, differences between nursing students and practicing nurses were reported in some aspects of hypothesis activation (Westfall et al., 1986) and in the amount of information obtained in identifying health problems (Broderick & Ammentorp, 1979). Corcoran (1986a, 1986b), reported differences between inexperienced and experienced hospice nurses in their approaches to planning care and in their ability to modify their approach depending on the complexity of the task. From comparisons between new graduates and experienced nurses, Benner (1984) reported development of expertise and other skilled performance along three dimensions: (a) progression from use of abstract principles as a basis for judgment to the use of past concrete experiences; (b) change in the subject's perception of the patient situation as a compilation of "equally relevant bits" of information to a perception of a complete whole, in which only selected bits are relevant; and (c) movement from detachment as an observer to full involvement in the situation. In three of the studies, the investigators anticipated statistically significant differences between the groups that were not detected (Broderick & Ammentorp, 1979; Corcoran, 1986a, 1986b; Westfall et al., 1986). The failure to find differences in each case may have been attributable to small sample sizes or insensitive measures.

Investigators have defined novice and expert differently and have focused on quite different components of clinical judgment performance. There is little cumulative information to date about the development of expertise in clinical judgment. The research does suggest that different processes are used by individual nurses depending on their level of expertise and on the demands of the task.

MEASURES OF CLINICAL JUDGMENT

An important aspect of teaching clinical judgment has been the availability of instruments useful for evaluating student performance. Research on the development and testing of measures of clinical judgment performance was quite limited both in quantity and scope. No studies were located in which investigators tested measures of actual clinical performance, although the use of observational measures such as rating scales and checklists has been recommended in the nursing literature for several years, and procedures for improving observer reliability have been reported (Lousteau et al., 1980). All instrument development studies that could be located were investigations of psychometric properties of five simulation tests assessing performance in clinical problem solving.

The most commonly used format for the simulation test has been the Patient Management Problem (PMP) originally developed by McGuire and her colleagues (McGuire & Babbot, 1967; McGuire & Solomon, 1971; McGuire, Solomon, & Bashook, 1975). The PMP is a written, branched simulation in which the examinees are presented with an initial description of a patient and are required to make judgments about what types of data to obtain and what types of actions to implement. After making their selections from a large array of possibilities, the examinees receive feedback about the consequences of their choices. The pathway through the problem is determined by the examinee's choices. Scoring is based largely on a comparison of the examinees' selection of either additional observations or interventions with the items deemed appropriate by a panel of experts. Hence, errors of commission and omission, together with a weighting of the seriousness of the errors, are used in the computation of the scores.

Psychometric evaluations of three simulation examinations using the PMP technique are reported in the nursing literature. Both deTornyay (1968a) and Dincher and Stidger (1976) developed single patient situations and evaluated their use with samples of undergraduate nursing students. Holzemer and associates (Farrand, Holzemer, & Schleutermann, 1982; Holzemer, Resnik, & Slichter, in press; Holzemer, Schleutermann, Farrand, & Miller, 1981) developed and evaluated three PMPs with a national sample of nurse practitioners and subsequent samples of nurses.

Two additional simulation techniques were used by McIntyre and associates and McLaughlin and associates (McIntyre, McDonald, Bailey, & Claus, 1972; McLaughlin, Carr, & Delucchi, 1980, 1981; McLaughlin, Cesa, Johnson, Lemons, Anderson, Larson, & Gibson, 1979; McLaughlin, Cesa, Johnson, Lemons, Anderson, Larson, Gibson, & Delucchi, 1979). Unlike the PMP, the simulations did not provide information and feedback contingent on the examinees' responses. McIntyre et al. evaluated some psychometric properties of their simulation test with a sample of undergraduate students, whereas McLaughlin and colleagues evaluated their instrument with a sample of physicians, nurse practitioners with and without master's degree preparation, public health nurses, and medical and nursing students.

Test–retest reliability was evaluated for three of the five simulation tests, and correlations ranged from low estimates in deTornyay's (1968a) study with a 4-week test–retest interval to "statistically significant" in the McIntyre et al. study (1972) with a 3-week interval, to surprisingly high ranges of .71 to .88 in the McLaughlin studies with a 60- to 90-day interval. The PMP used in the Holzemar studies and the clinical simulation test in the McLaughlin studies each had a high degree of internal consistency reliability (Holzemer & McLaughlin, in press). The interpretation of both test–retest reliability and internal consistency reliability on these linear, branching tests has been debatable.

The approach to content validation in all studies was the use of an expert panel that determined the weighting of the choices of observations and interventions as essential, nonessential, and inappropriate. Because this weighting was used as the basis for subsequent scoring, the selection of the panel was extremely important. A clear strength of the McLaughlin studies was the careful selection of panels, which were chosen according to strict criteria from a national sample of experts.

Construct validity was evaluated using the known group method in four studies with the following comparisons: between nursing students and other students (deTornyay, 1968a), between student nurses in an experimental curriculum designed to improve problem solving and those in a traditional curriculum (McIntyre et al., 1972), between nurse clinicians and students (McLaughlin et al., 1980, 1981), and among groups of nurse clinicians with varying levels of preparation and experience (Farrand et al., 1982; McLaughlin, Cesa, Johnson, Lemons, Anderson, Larson, & Gibson, 1979; McLaughlin, Cesa, Johnson, Lemons, Anderson, Larson, Gibson, & Delucchi, 1979). In all comparisons, support for construct validity was claimed on the basis of statistically significant differences between the groups in the predicted direction.

The extent to which the PMP and other simulation tests measure the clinical judgment performance that would occur in actual clinical practice has been estimated in several ways, with discouraging results. Holzemer et al. (1981) found very low correlations between PMP scores and clinical performance measured by self-evaluation, colleague evaluation, and audit. In fact, scores on a multiple choice examination of knowledge were correlated more highly with the clinical performance measures than were the PMP scores. In a later study of 17 nurse practitioners, Holzemer, Resnik, and Slichter (in press) found that a chart audit and observation data were correlated significantly with one another, but neither were correlated with the clinical simulation scores. In contrast, Dincher and Stidger (1976), with their sample of 11 students, found a significant correlation between rank order of scores on the PMP and clinical instructor's rank ordering of performance in clinical practice. The failure to find significant correlations between clinical performance measures and clinical simulations has been a fairly consistent finding in studies of physicians and medical students (Goran, Williamson, & Gonnella, 1973; Page & Fielding, 1980) and may have been a function of poor criterion measures, invalidity of the PMP, or a combination of both.

To examine further the issue of the quality of a criterion measure in criterion-related validity, Holzemer and McLaughlin (in press) explored the relationship between the PMP used in the earlier Holzemer studies and the clinical simulation tests used in the McLaughlin studies. There was a positive relationship between the PMP and two of the four simulations. These findings stimulated Holzemer (1986) to do additional analyses in order to assess the nature of problem solving strategies used in response to PMP simulations. Data from the original studies of one PMP were analyzed using correlational procedures and factor analysis. Three factors emerged as predictive of performance: data gathering, laboratory performance, and patient education.

On the the basis of these few studies, it cannot be concluded that simulation methods provide valid measures of performance in clinical judgment. Because of their questionable validity, Holzemer et al. (in press) recommended that nurse educators use caution in adopting simulations for purposes of evaluation.

INSTRUCTIONAL METHODS

In recent years, a number of theoretical articles have appeared in which the authors have attempted to derive appropriate teaching strategies from the descriptive literature on general problem solving (Yeaw, 1979) and on clinical decision making (Jenkins, 1985). Although there are numerous anecdotal descriptions of successful approaches to teaching clinical judgment, only five studies (Aspinall, 1979; deTornyay, 1968b; Hamdi & Hutelmyer, 1970; Mitchell & Atwood, 1975; Tanner, 1982) have been identified that included systematic evaluation of strategies for teaching clinical judgment.

In two of the studies, researchers investigated what might be considered "aids" to assessment and diagnosis rather than teaching strategies intended to produce a generalizable improvement in clinical judgment. Aspinall (1979) tested the effectiveness of using decision trees to improve diagnostic accuracy. Experimental group nurses were given a set of binary decision trees to enable them to use information systematically and to determine if characteristics of each condition were present. The experimental group performed significantly better than the control group. In a second study, Hamdi and Hutelmyer (1970) examined the effectiveness of using a structured assessment guide in improving nurses' abilities to identify pertinent nursing care problems. There were no differences between the experimental group and the control group on number of valid problems identified in the assessment of 10 patients, but the experimental group was able to provide a significantly greater number of reasons substantiating the problems than the control group. One could draw a rather obvious conclusion from these studies: if nurses were told what to look for and how to interpret the data obtained, they were able to make relevant observations and to interpret the observations appropriately.

In three additional studies, researchers examined the effectiveness of theoretically based teaching methods on improving clinical judgment abilities of baccalaureate nursing students. Both the teaching methods and outcome measures were quite diverse. DeTornyay (1968b) designed an experimental teaching strategy to assist students in the discovery of concepts and principles. Performance was measured on a written patient management problem. There were no significant main effects from the experimental teaching strategy.

Mitchell and Atwood (1975) compared a group of beginning nursing students who were taught problem-oriented charting with a group taught traditional charting. Although the experimental group identified significantly more patient problems in their clinical charting, there were no differences between the groups in the number of patient problems identified from a written patient situation.

Tanner (1982) designed an experimental teaching method based on descriptive studies of diagnostic reasoning processes. The experimental strategy differed from the traditional approach in two respects: (a) the organization of content to facilitate activation of diagnostic hypotheses, which was presumed to be a central activity in diagnostic reasoning, and (b) practice, through written exercises, in generating and testing diagnostic hypotheses. Scores on diagnostic ability were derived from verbal responses to five videotaped simulations. There were no significant main effects from the experimental treatment.

There are several explanations for the failure to find significant generalizable improvement in clinical judgment following a teaching intervention. In each of the studies, the experimental treatment has been extremely short, from an average of 4.5 hours in deTornyay's (1968b), to 15 hours in Tanner's (1982), to a term in Mitchell and Atwood's (1975). Instruction in processes as complex as clinical judgment probably require far more time to modify performance. Instrumentation is also an issue as the search for valid measures of clinical judgment performance continues. Although the results of these few studies are discouraging, it is premature to abandon hope that effective approaches to teaching clinical judgment can be discovered.

CORRELATES OF CLINICAL JUDGMENT PERFORMANCE

In an effort to explore ways in which performance in clinical judgment may be improved, several investigators have conducted correlational studies, searching for factors that may be associated with clinical judgment proficiency. Among these factors are level of education and years of nursing experience, the critical thinking abilities of students or nurses, discipline membership (e.g., nurse, physician, health administrator), the type of conceptual model used in the undergraduate nursing curriculum, and the personality profile of the student.

There were six studies in which investigators examined the relationship between clinical judgment ability, and education and experience. These studies were strikingly similar in both methods and findings and unlike most other areas of clinical judgment research, they provided clear evidence of building on prior work. In four studies investigators used a series of filmed patient situations originally developed by Verhonick and associates (Davis, 1972, 1974; Frederickson & Mayer, 1977; Verhonick, Nichols, Glor, & McCarthy, 1968). Subjects responded to each situation by listing pertinent observations, identifying nursing actions and providing reasons for those actions; scores were derived from a comparison of subjects' responses with those of a panel of experts. In three of the four studies (Davis, 1972, 1974; Verhonick et al., 1968), performance was related positively to the academic degree held. There was also a generally negative relationship between performance and years of nursing experience in subjects with more than six years of experience, although the finding was not consistent in all measures, nor in all groups. Frederickson and Mayer (1977) argued that there was no relationship between education and performance but provided no data to support their contention.

A positive relationship between performance and academic degree was reported by two additional investigators who used somewhat different methods. Del Bueno (1983) used a newly developed series of 12 patient situations to elicit the same three responses requested in the Verhonick et al. (1968) instrument. Aspinall (1976) used a single written case study, requesting subjects to identify possible causes for a patient's condition. Both investigators reported that nurses with a baccalaureate degree performed better than nurses with either a diploma or an associate degree. Although the use of T-tests for multiple comparisons in the Aspinall study increased the likelihood of chance findings, the consistency of this finding in several studies supports its veracity. Aspinall also found a decline in performance in nurses with more than 10 years of experience. That there was not a decline in performance with experience in the del Bueno study may have been a function of treating experience as a dichotomous variable.

In four studies the relationship between performance on a measure of clinical judgment and performance on a test of general problem-solving ability was evaluated. Although the investigators used quite different measures of clinical judgment, three employed the Watson Glaser Critical Thinking Appraisal (WGCTA) (Watson & Glaser, 1952) as the measure of general problem-solving ability. In studies of undergraduate students (Matthews & Gaul, 1979; Tanner, 1982), graduate students (Matthews & Gaul, 1979), and nurse practitioners (Holzemer & McLaughlin, in press), there consistently was no significant relationship between the performance in clinical judgment and the overall score or subscale scores on the WGCTA. Gordon (1980) found no relationship among graduate students between scores in diagnostic ability and scores on either the Graduate Record Examination or the Miller Analogies Test.

Comparison among disciplines on aspects of clinical judgment was the focus of two programs of studies (Hansen & Thomas, 1968a, 1968b, 1969; McLaughlin, Cesa, Johnson, Lemons, Anderson, Larson, & Gibson, 1979a; McLaughlin, Cesa, Johnson, Lemons, Anderson, Larson, Gibson, & Delucchi, 1979b; Thomas & Hansen, 1966, 1969). Hansen and Thomas compared four professional groups, health officers, public health staff nurses and supervisors, and nursing faculty, and two undergraduate nursing student groups, before and after public health nursing experience. They found differences in judgments for both decision areas tested, the assignment of priorities for home visits and the importance of advising medical care. McLaughlin and associates found no differences in proficiency between nurse practitioners and physicians on two simulation tests. The physicians' practice style was less psychosocial, but not more pathophysiological, than that of the nurse practitioners.

Within this category of research were two one-of-a-kind studies in which investigators examined two additional correlates of clinical judgment performance. DeBack (1981) found no relationship between senior nursing students' ability to formulate nursing diagnoses and the type of curriculum model. Koehne-Kaplan and Tilden (1976) examined the relationship between personality type and clinical judgment skills. There was no significant relationship between the two measures. The theoretical bases for predicted relationships in both of these studies were somewhat weak; moreover, the measures of clinical judgment in both studies and the categorization of schools in the DeBack investigation may not have been sufficiently sensitive to detect individual differences.

ISSUES AND ASSUMPTIONS

Several methodological and conceptual issues applied to a large portion of this research literature. The most frequent methodological problems were in the areas of sampling and instrumentation. Predominant were small convenience samples drawn from volunteers in one or two institutions. Although this may have been appropriate for exploratory research, the willingness on the part of investigators to make generalizations to populations not sampled was troublesome. Notable exceptions to this problem were in the work of Benner (1984), DeBack (1981), Holzemer and associates (Farrand et al., 1982; Holzemer et al., 1981), and McLaughlin and associates (1979b, 1980, 1981).

The problems with instrumentation are related to the heavy reliance on simulation as a means of assessing performance in clinical judgment, as an outcome measure of instructional effectiveness, or as the method to elicit subject response for describing processes of clinical judgment. There are two major concerns with use of simulations: The tasks may not be representative of clinical judgment tasks, and the responses elicited may not be like those that would occur in actual practice.

Most of the simulations have required that the subject read a brief description or view a videotaped vignette of a client experiencing some problem; subjects were then required to identify the problem or decide on appropriate nursing actions and their priority. The situations portrayed were usually few in number; most studies have only one, and could not have been representative of either the vast array of content of possible health problems nor of the structure of situations that may promote use of different kinds of clinical judgment processes. The kinds of clinical judgment required to assist clients in health promotion, to establish plans for next stages of rehabilitation, to respond to emergency situations, or to interact with a family in a supportive and therapeutic manner have not been investigated. The lack of generalizability of the simulations to the range of problem-solving, decision-making, or other judgment situations seldom is acknowleged.

The reliance on simulation is also problematic from the standpoint of representativeness of responses. The extent to which subjects' responses are valid representations of their performance in practice continues to be a matter of controversy, despite efforts in the measurement literature (Holzemer et al., 1981; in press) to address this question. Therefore, descriptions of the clinical judgment processes, identified educational or individual correlates of clinical judgment performance, and reported effectiveness of instructional methods may not be generalizable to performance in actual clinical practice.

As most investigators have realized, there are few alternatives to the use of simulations, to measure performance in clinical judgment and, hence, for assessing instructional effectiveness. It is obviously premature to abandon efforts in simulation, particularly because the approach offers an opportunity to examine the performance of several subjects on the same task, but the method needs to be augmented with additional measures of performance in clinical judgment.

In addition to the methodological issues, there were several problems related to the theoretical contribution of the research literature. Many of the studies, particularly in the area of correlates to clinical judgment performance, were either atheoretical or weak conceptually. As a result, little understanding can be gleaned from findings of positive correlations between two or more variables. Very few of the studies were designed to test a theory, although one or more theoretical frameworks were described as background in nearly one third. Even when investigators described several theoretical perspectives, there was little evidence of using any theory to guide either the research questions or the design of the study. Consequently, from a theoretical perspective very little can be concluded about the processes of clinical judgment or about ways to teach and evaluate students in their use of these processes.

Underlying much of this research literature appears to be the assumption that there is a single process or set of procedures of clinical judgment that can be described, measured, and taught. Henderson (1982) recently has questioned this assumption in her analysis of the terminology regarding the nursing process, suggesting that different types of nursing care require different types of processes, such as intuitive judgment, and that not all of nursing practice could be described as an analytic, problem-solving activity. In most of the studies there has been a search for the single underlying process, or a method to teach the single process or to measure it. That there may not be a single process is suggested in the work of investigators studying novice–expert differences (Benner, 1984; Broderick & Ammentorp, 1979; Corcoran, 1986a; Westfall et al., 1986) and in studies in which more than one patient situation is presented (Holzemer, in press) or where situations are varied systematically (Corcoran, 1986b).

FUTURE RESEARCH DIRECTIONS

The research related to teaching clinical judgment is a somewhat amorphous collection of studies only loosely related to one another. There is little evidence of a cumulative effort in research. With the diversity in theoretical perspectives and the lack of clear direction in replication, refinement, or extension of prior work, little can be concluded about the processes of clinical judgment nor about effective ways to teach and evaluate students in their use of those processes. It is clear from the correlational literature that there is some relationship between education and the ability to make clinical judgments on a simulation test. There is also increasing evidence that different processes are used depending on the level of expertise and the nature of the patient situation. There is little guidance in terms of what to teach or how to teach it for educators wishing to improve the students' performance in clinical judgment.

There are some encouraging trends. Studies published in more recent years and those in press show increasing strength in their conceptualization and increasing relevance of the method for testing the theory. There is also promise for greater cumulative efforts in that several investigators are continuing to develop research programs. For continued development of the knowledge base related to teaching clinical judgment, these trends need to be supported.

Methodological inquiry for research on clinical judgment is needed. The recent introduction of the phenomenological approach to the study of clinical judgment greatly augments the use of simulations and verbal protocol analysis. It is clear that a combination of methods and an increased understanding of their strengths and limitations are needed for research in this complex area.

In the area of processes of clinical judgment, research is needed on virtually all components from observation to patient management. Continued study of differences between novice and expert performance is important both for its potential contribution to knowledge about processes and also for its potential to guide instructional decisions. An area of investigation fundamental to all other research on clinical judgment is a description of the nature of nursing tasks and an understanding of the ways in which these characteristics influence use of judgment strategies.

Research on teaching and measuring clinical judgment, for both practical and theoretical reasons, needs greater emphasis. Investigators examining processes of clinical judgment have suggested the adoption of one or more approaches to teaching that warrant systematic investigation. Instruction in formal decision theory, heuristic strategies such as hypothesis generation and testing used in diagnosis, and learning to attend to important aspects of a situation through working with experts all have been suggested as appropriate teaching strategies needing study.

The search for correlates of clinical judgment performance has been largely unsuccessful. This likely will continue to be the case until the construct of clinical judgment is better defined and the processes employed are better understood. It is not a high priority area for continued research, except to the extent that identifying correlates assists in developing and refining theories of clinical judgment.

REFERENCES

Aspinall, M. J. (1976). Nursing diagnosis—The weak link. *Nursing Outlook, 24*, 433, 437.

Aspinall, M. J. (1979). Use of a decision tree to improve accuracy of diagnosis. *Nursing Research, 28*, 182–185.

Baumann, A., & Bourbonnais, F. (1982). Nursing decision making in critical care areas. *Journal of Advanced Nursing, 7*, 435–446.

Benner, P. (1984). *From novice to expert: Power and excellence in nursing practice*. Palo Alto, CA: Addison-Wesley.

Benner, P., & Wrubel, J. (1982). Skilled clinical knowledge: The value of perceptual awareness. *Nursing Educator, 7*(3), 11–17.

Broderick, M. E., & Ammentorp, W. (1979). Information structures: An analysis of nursing performance. *Nursing Research, 28*, 106–110.

Bruner, J. S., Goodnow, J. J., & Austin, G. A. (1956). *A study of thinking*. New York: Wiley.

Cianfrani, K. L. (1984). The influence of amounts and relevance of data on identifying health problems. In M. J. Kim, G. K. McFarland, & A. M. McLane (Eds.), *Classifications of nursing diagnoses: Proceedings of the Fifth National Conference* (pp. 150–161). St. Louis: Mosby.

Corcoran, S. (1986a). Planning by expert and novice nurses in cases of varying complexity. *Research in Nursing and Health, 9*, 155–162.

Corcoran, S. (1986b). Task complexity and nursing expertise as factors in decision making. *Nursing Research, 35*, 107–112.

Davis, B. G. (1972). Clinical expertise as a function of educational preparation. *Nursing Research, 21*, 530–534.

Davis, B. G. (1974). Effect of levels of nursing education on patient care: A replication. *Nursing Research, 23*, 150–155.

DeBack, V. (1981). The relationship between senior nursing students' ability to formulate nursing diagnoses and the curriculum model. *Advances in Nursing Science, 3*(3), 51–66.

del Bueno, D. J. (1983). Doing the right thing: Nurses' ability to make clinical decisions. *Nurse Educator, 8*(3), 7–11.

deTornyay, R. (1968a). Measuring problem-solving skills by means of the simulated clinical nursing problem test. *Journal of Nursing Education, 5*(8), 3–8, 34–35.

deTornyay, R. (1968b). The effect of an experimental teaching strategy on problem solving abilities of sophomore nursing students. *Nursing Research, 17*, 108–114.

Dincher, J. R., & Stidger, S. L. (1976). Evaluation of a written simulation format for clinical nursing judgment: A pilot study. *Nursing Research, 25*, 280–285.

Farrand, L., Holzemer, W. L., & Schleutermann, J. A. (1982). A study on construct validity: Simulations as a measure of nurse practitioner problem-solving skills. *Nursing Research, 31*, 37–42.

Frederickson, K., & Mayer, G. G. (1977). Problem solving skills. What effect does education have? *American Journal of Nursing, 77*, 1167–1169.

Gebbie, K., & Lavin, M. A. (Eds.). (1975). *Classification of nursing diagnoses: Proceedings of the First National Conference.* St. Louis: Mosby.

Goran, M. J., Williamson, J. W., & Gonella, J. S. (1973). The validity of patient management problems. *Journal of Medical Education, 48*, 171–177.

Gordon, M. (1980). Predictive strategies in diagnostic tasks. *Nursing Research, 29*, 39–45.

Grier, M. R. (1976). Decision making about patient care. *Nursing Research, 25*, 105–110.

Grier, M. (1984). Information processing in nursing practice. In H. H. Werley & J. J. Fitzpatrick (Eds.), *Annual Review of Nursing Research* (Vol. 2) (pp. 265–287). New York: Springer Publishing.

Hamdi, M. E., & Hutelmyer, C. M. (1970). A study of the effectiveness of an assessment tool in the identification of nursing care problems. *Nursing Research, 19*, 354–359.

Hammond, K. R. (1966). Clinical inference in nursing: II. A psychologist's viewpoint. *Nursing Research, 15*, 27–38.

Hammond, K. R., Kelly, K. J., Castellan, N. J., Schneider, R. J., & Vancini, M. (1966). Clinical inference in nursing: Use of information-seeking strategies by nurses. *Nursing Research, 15*, 330–336.

Hammond, K. R., Kelly, K. J., Schneider, R. J., & Vancini, M. (1966a). Clinical inference in nursing: Analyzing cognitive tasks representatave of nursing problems. *Nursing Research, 15*, 134–138.

Hammond, K. R., Kelly, K. J., Schneider, R. J., & Vancini, M. (1966b). Clinical inference in nursing: Information units used. *Nursing Research, 15*, 236–243.

Hammond, K. R., Kelly, K. J., Schneider, R. J., & Vancini, M. (1967). Clinical inference in nursing: Revising judgments. *Nursing Research, 16*, 38–45.

Hansen, A. C., & Thomas, D. B. (1968a). A conceptualization of decision making: Its application to a study of role and situation-related difference in priority decisions. *Nursing Research, 17*, 436–443.

Hansen, A. C., & Thomas, D. B. (1968b). Role group differences in judging the importance of advising medical care. *Nursing Research, 17*, 525–532.

Hansen, A. C., & Thomas, D. B. (1969). Differences and changes in decision judgments within two role groups. *Nursing Research, 18*, 333–338.

Henderson, V. (1982). The nursing process—Is the title right? *Journal of Advanced Nursing, 7*, 103–109.

Holzemer, W. L. (1986). The structure of problem-solving in simulations. *Nursing Research, 35*, 231–236.

Holzemer, W. L., & McLaughlin, F. E. (in press). Concurrent validity of clinical simulations. *Western Journal of Nursing Research.*

Holzemer, W. L., Resnik, B., & Slichter, M. (in press). Criterion-related validity of a clinical simulation. *Journal of Nursing Education.*

Holzemer, W. L., Schleutermann, J. A., Farrand, L., & Miller, A. G. (1981). A validation study: Simulations as a measure of nurse practitioners' problem solving skills. *Nursing Research, 30*, 139–144.

Jenkins, H. M. (1985). Improving clinical decision making in nursing. *Journal of Nursing Education, 24*, 242–245.

Kelly, K. (1966). Clinical inference in nursing: I. A nurse's viewpoint. *Nursing Research, 15*, 23–26.

Kim, M. J., McFarland, G. K., & McLane, A. M. (Eds.) (1984). *Classification of nursing diagnosis: Proceedings of the Fifth National Conference.* St. Louis: Mosby.

Kim, M. J., & Moritz, D. A. (Eds.) (1982). *Classification of nursing diagnosis: Proceedings of the Third and Fourth National Conferences.* New York: McGraw-Hill.

Koehne-Kaplan, N. S., & Tilden, V. P. (1976). The process of clinical judgment in nursing practice: The component of personality. *Nursing Research, 25*, 268–272.

Loustau, A., Lentz, M., Lee, K., McKenna, M., Hirako, S., Walker, W. F., & Goldsmith, J. W. (1980). Evaluating students' clinical performance: Using videotape to establish rater reliability. *Journal of Nursing Education, 19*(7), 10–17.

Matthews, C. A., & Gaul, A. L. (1979). Nursing diagnosis from the perspective of concept attainment and critical thinking. *Advances in Nursing Science, 2*(1), 17–26.

McGuire, C. H. (1985). Medical problem-solving: A critique of the literature. *Journal of Medical Education, 60*, 587–595.

McGuire, C. H., & Babbott, D. (1967). Simulation technique in the measurement of problem solving skills. *Journal of Educational Measurement, 4*, 1–10.

McGuire, C. H., & Solomon, L. M. (1971). *Clinical simulations: Selected problems in patient management.* New York: Appleton-Century-Crofts.

McGuire, C. H., Solomon, L. M., & Bashook, P. G. (1975). *Construction and use of written simulations.* New York: Psychological Corporation.

McIntyre, H. N., McDonald, F. J., Bailey, J. T., & Claus, K. K. (1972). A simulated clinical nursing test. *Nursing Research, 21*, 429–435.

McLaughlin, F. E., Carr, J., & Delucchi, K. (1980). Selected psychometric properties of two clinical simulation tests. *Journal of Medical Education, 55*, 375–376.

McLaughlin, F. E., Carr, J., & Delucchi, K. (1981). Measurement properties of clinical simulation tests: Hypertension and chronic obstructive pulmonary disease. *Nursing Research, 30*, 5–9.

McLaughlin, F. E., Cesa, T., Johnson, H., Lemons, M., Anderson, S., Larson,

P., & Gibson, J. (1979a). Nurses' and physicians' performance on clinical simulation test: Hypertension. *Research in Nursing and Health, 2*, 61–72.

McLaughlin, F. E., Cesa, T., Johnson, H., Lemons, M., Anderson, S., Larson, P., Gibson, J., & Delucchi, K. (1979b). Nurse practitioners', public health nurses', and physicians' performance on clinical simulation test: COPD. *Western Journal of Nursing Research, 2*, 21–29.

Mitchell, P. H., & Atwood, J. (1975). Problem-oriented recording as a teaching-learning tool. *Nursing Research, 24*, 99–103.

National League for Nursing. (1983). *Criteria for the evaluation of baccalaureate and higher degree programs in nursing.* New York: Author.

Newell, A., & Simon, H. (1972). *Human problem solving.* Englewood Cliffs, NJ: Prentice-Hall.

Page, G. G., & Fielding, D. W. (1980). Performance on PMPs and performance in practice: Are they related? *Journal of Medical Education, 55*, 529–537.

Phillips, L. R., & Rempusheski, V. F. (1985). Diagnosing and intervening for elder abuse and neglect: An empirically generated decision-making model. *Nursing Research, 34*, 134–139.

Pyles, S. H., & Stern, P. N. (1983). Discovery of nursing gestalt in critical care nursing: The importance of the gray gorilla syndrome. *Image: The Journal of Nursing Scholarship, 15*(2), 51–57.

Santora, D. (1980). *Conceptual frameworks used in baccalaureate and master's degree curricula.* New York: National League for Nursing.

Tanner, C. A. (1982). Instruction in the diagnostic process: An experimental study. In M. J. Kim & D. Moritz (Eds.), *Classification of nursing diagnoses: Proceedings of the Third and Fourth National Conferences* (pp. 145–152). New York: McGraw-Hill.

Tanner, C. A., & Lindeman, C. A. (in press). Research in nursing education: Priorities and assumptions. *Journal of Nursing Education.*

Thomas, D. B., & Hansen, A. C. (1966). Role group differences in assignment of priorities: A variable perspective interpretation. *Nursing Research, 15*, 12–19.

Thomas, D. B., & Hansen, A. C. (1969). Multiple discriminant analysis of public health nursing decision responses. *Nursing Research, 18*, 145–153.

Verhonick, P. J., Nichols, G. A., Glor, B. A. K., & McCarthy, R. T. (1968). I came, I saw, I responded: Nursing observation and action survey. *Nursing Research, 17*, 38–44.

Watson, G., & Glaser, E. M. (1952). *Watson–Glaser critical thinking appraisal manual.* Yonkers-on-Hudson, NY: World Book.

Westfall, U. E., Tanner, C. A., Putzier, D. J., & Padrick, K. P. (1986). Clinical inferences in nursing: A preliminary analysis of cognitive strategies. *Research in Nursing and Health, 9*, 269–277.

Yeaw, E. M. J. (1979). Problem solving as a method of teaching: Strategies in classroom and clinical teaching. *Journal of Nursing Education, 18*(7), 16–22.

PART IV

Research on
the Profession of Nursing

Chapter 8

Leadership in Nursing

JOANNE COMI MCCLOSKEY
COLLEGE OF NURSING
UNIVERSITY OF IOWA
AND
MARILYN T. MOLEN
BACHELOR OF ARTS IN NURSING PROGRAM
METROPOLITAN STATE UNIVERSITY

CONTENTS

A crisis in leadership is one of the greatest challenges facing the nursing profession today. Within our health care system we now have a work force of 1.6 million nurses in settings ranging from large corporate institutions to private practice. Scientific breakthroughs and innovative technology have extended the boundaries of health care to unlimited potential. As a result, the knowledge and skill necessary for effective nursing care is greater than ever before. Technological advances and a concomitant concern for cost containment have placed the health care delivery system in a state of turmoil, and, as the largest health care discipline, nursing is facing major changes in education and practice. As never before, nursing needs leaders who are competent, flexible, politically savvy, willing to accept diversity, and able to energize others to adapt to change.

Leadership is the process of influencing people to accomplish goals, whereas management is moving an organization toward achievement of its goals. Leadership is not management, but it is hoped, indeed necessary, that managers are leaders. Key concepts that comprise leadership include influence, communication, group process, goal attainment, and motivation. Recent leadership theory indicates that assessment of the situation and adjustment of style to fit the situation are key elements of a successful leader (Fiedler, Mahar, & Chemars, 1977; Hersey & Blanchard, 1982; Reddin, 1970). Adjusting one's style to meet expectations and abilities of the followers is perhaps the biggest challenge for any leader. When the expectations and abilities of the followers do not match the goals of the organization, the leader's task is even more difficult. In this important area, little direction exists for nurses. What can research tell us about leadership in nursing?

The method for this research review incorporated both computer and manual searches. A MEDLARS computer search was conducted for the years 1966 to 1983 using the descriptors of *leadership* and *nursing*. A second MEDLARS search was done for the years 1978 to 1984 with the descriptors *leadership, nursing*, and *role*. Manual searches were completed of the *Cumulative Index to Nursing and Allied Health Literature*, 1982 to 1984; of dissertation abstracts under management and health indexes, 1968 to 1984; and of reference lists obtained from articles and books on leadership. Several additional sources known to the authors from their previous work were checked. Over 200 citations were found, with the vast majority being opinion or theoretical pieces. In reviewing the literature on leadership the following criteria were used for inclusion in this report: (a) research-based, (b) relevant to leadership in nursing, and (c) written in English. Using these criteria, 58 studies were found.

It should be noted that the subject of leadership in nursing is not one with easily identifiable boundaries. While it is not difficult to locate research reports with leadership in the titles, there may have been relevant studies without our descriptors as headings. These would have been omitted from this review unless they had been picked up through our manual search.

A review of the dissertation abstracts yielded a number of relevant studies, particularly from the mid to late 1970s. However, because of time and cost to purchase and review the microfiche copies, we did not include them in our review. In the final analysis, then, this is a review of published research reports that are presented in four categories: defining leadership, predicting leadership, leadership development, and leadership effectiveness. Evolving from a content analysis of the research that was reviewed, the categories are not mutually exclusive, although each study is discussed in only one category. From our review, it is apparent that leadership has been talked about more than studied. This chapter, therefore, represents a beginning attempt to organize the research in this area into meaningful categories for analysis.

DEFINING LEADERSHIP

Much of the early research on leadership consisted of case study analyses of nurses who have made a substantial contribution to the profession. In a classic set of historical case studies, for instance, Teresa E. Christy described the characteristics and contributions of seven well-known nursing leaders: Lavina Dock (1969c); Annie Warbuton Goodrich (1970b); M. Adelaide Nutting (1969a); Sophia F. Palmer (1975); Isabel Hampton Robb (1969b); Isabel Maitland Stewart (1969d); and Lillian D. Wald (1970a). The characteristics of these early nurse leaders varied, including personal attributes such as being dignified, courageous, warmhearted, visionary, intellectual, patient, enthusiastic, energetic, risk taking, determined, decisive, hardworking, and committed. Their accomplishments as change agents, builders, and innovators also varied. They started schools of nursing, professional organizations, nursing publications, and deanships; they made legislative changes, changes in nursing practice, and changes in nursing education. Each leader was influential and each contributed substantially to the development of nursing.

Three case studies of contemporary nurse leaders are available: Hildegard Peplau (Sills, 1978), Rozella Schlotfeldt (Corona, 1981), and Margretta Styles (Langford, 1983). These leaders are recognized for their contributions to the scholarly and academic traditions of nursing.

The case studies were published in practice journals and included little detail as to methodology. Two of the latter studies were reports of interviews. Christy did not approach her historical studies with a set of research questions. Rather, she chronicled the life and activities of these figures. The case study approach was an appropriate methodology for this topic, especially if applied with more rigor.

Leadership also has been defined by developing profiles of nurses who occupied positions of leadership. A typical descriptive study was reported by Brimmer, Skoner, Pender, Williams, Lleming, and Werley (1983). They conducted a 2-year survey to determine education and employment characteristics of nurses with doctoral degrees. Although leadership was not the focus and was not defined beyond holding the doctorate, the study was based on the premise that leadership in nursing required that attention be given to professional socialization of nurses at the doctoral level.

Deans of schools or colleges of nursing have been recognized as a prominent leadership group. The most complete description of who nursing deans are and what they do was provided by the American Association of Colleges of Nursing (Johnson, 1983). This study was a replication of a 1978 survey of social work deans. Findings indicated that, compared with social work deans, nursing deans more often were women, younger and with less experience, less likely to have a doctorate, published less, and more likely to head up undergraduate-only programs. Examining the dean's role from the perspective of a minority group, George (1982) described eight black deans, their responsibilities, and their perceptions of the decanal role. She recommended an emphasis on mentoring, networking, and career development programs to facilitate the socialization of an educator to the role of dean.

Some studies have been conducted to ascertain nurses' perception of leadership. For example, in a small pilot investigation Davidson (1968) collected nursing students' perceptions of what activities constituted leadership in nursing practice. From this unsophisticated study, she concluded that there was not a clear, consistent definition of leadership among nursing students. Inconsistent perceptions also were found in a survey of 145 sets of chief operating officers and directors of nursing in hospitals (Survey, 1977). Chief operating officers were more likely to view the director as nurse than as director. The author provided few details of the methodology.

Some researchers have described what nurses actually did in their leadership roles. Jones and Jones (1979) grouped activities of eight head nurses according to Mintzberg's roles of the manager, and Demi and Miles (1984) applied leadership and nursing process concepts to responses of nurses during a disaster situation. Baker (1981) focused her investigation on the leadership behaviors of academic department heads to determine their involvement in three areas: school, scholarship, and profession. Incomplete reporting was a problem in each of the three studies.

Characteristics, roles, and responsibilities of the contemporary hospital nurse administrator were examined in a survey of nurses holding membership in the American Hospital Association's American Society of Nursing Service Administrators (Aydelotte, 1984). Results demonstrated that, in contrast to the 1960s, the scope of the leadership role of today's nurse executive has expanded.

The studies just reviewed give us a profile of characteristics, activities, and behaviors of nurse leaders. Ranging from studies of deans, doctorally prepared nurses, and nurse administrators to studies of head nurses, disaster nurses, and senior nursing students, the focus of these descriptive efforts has varied widely. Findings suggest that leadership consists of personal as well as functional and situational elements. Although few generalizations can be drawn, it does appear that the effective leader has energy, commitment, and communication and change skills. Several of the studies in this section lack complete reporting.

PREDICTING LEADERSHIP

Personality characteristics and personal qualities indicating leadership potential or leadership success have been the focus of several studies. For example, Kelly (1974) used four personality tests to determine whether he could predict which staff nurses would be promoted to assistant head nurse. Results of the well-designed study indicated that capacity for status, a "feminine" attitude, and poise were the best predictors of promotion. In another well-designed study, Gilbert (1975) used the California Psychological Inventory (Gough, 1969) to examine leadership potential of graduate nursing students. Personality traits that distinguished the leaders from nonleaders were: dominance, aggressiveness, ambition, high capacity to attain status, poise, self-confidence, tolerance for others' views, high need to achieve, a well-ordered mind, sensitivity to others' needs, and flexibility.

To determine the relationship between leadership effectiveness and personality characteristics, Gluck and Charter (1980) studied staff nurses in a Veterans Administration (VA) hospital using the Cattel 16 Personality Factor Questionnaire (Cattell, Eber, & Tatsuoka, 1974). Less experienced nurses were more assertive, whereas the experienced nurses were more submissive, dependent, conforming, and easily led. Although the authors concluded that the personality traits of warmth and assertiveness were needed to be an effective leader, they did not actually measure leader effectiveness.

Hanson and Chater (1983) used a test of personality, Holland's Vocational Preference Inventory (1978), along with a measure of management interest, the Strong–Campbell Inventory (Campbell, 1977), to test the proposition that women in nursing sought roles that permitted the expression of their personalities. Responses from nursing graduate students indicated that those with management interests were more practical minded, sociable, conforming, dominant, expressive, and had more occupational interest. Unfortunately, the authors did not investigate whether nurses with management interests actually became managers.

In a large-scale investigation, Schwirian used academic achievement as the predictor of leadership success. Schwirian (1977, 1978, 1979) compared ratings of leadership in two groups of nurses: those identified as most promising by their academic achievement in nursing school and those not identified as such. Supervisor evaluations were obtained by asking each nurse to supply his or her supervisor's name and address, a procedure that may have contributed to the low response rate of 30%. The graduates identified as most promising had higher mean supervisor ratings than those graduates not so designated. Findings implied that demonstrated potential for leadership in school was a good indication of future performance. One result of this large study was the development of the 6-D Scale of Nursing Performance, part of which measures leadership.

Finally, Sheridan and Vredenburgh (1978) examined situation variables to determine which were most significant in predicting the leadership behavior of head nurses. Leadership behavior of head nurses was rated by subordinates using the Leader Behavior Description Questionnaire (Stogdill, 1963). Results indicated that staff turnover was the most important predictor of the head nurse's leadership behavior; however, the investigators admitted that this finding could indicate a converse relationship, namely that head nurses' leadership behavior influenced staff turnover.

In short, a review of the scanty investigative efforts concerned with predicting leadership in nursing indicates that most of this research has focused on the relationship between personality characteristics and leadership. Other areas that deserve attention include management interest, academic achievement, and situational factors. Longitudinal methodologies would lead to more conclusive findings.

LEADERSHIP DEVELOPMENT

Knowing what leadership skills are needed in various situations and being able to identify potential leaders are the prerequisites to leadership development. Only eight studies are reviewed in this area. Six are concerned with career advancement and two focus on strategies for leadership development.

Career advancement in the practice setting was examined in two studies. Knudson (1968) used a stratified sample of staff-level public health nurses, supervisors, and administrators from 13 public health agencies to identify factors related to their interest in advancing into administrative positions. She found statistically significant associations between interest in career advancement and (a) career orientation toward work, (b) influence toward higher education by the subject's mother or significant others, (c) age, (d) baccalaureate education, (e) willingness to take a risk on taking a job, and (f) viewing chances for promotion as favorable. Friss (1983) studied directors of nursing from 150 hospitals in California to determine their career style, career development, and career longevity. She found that the most important predictor of organizational commitment was professional commitment. It was difficult to interpret her findings, however, because the report was incomplete and somewhat unclear.

Researchers examined socialization and career advancement in the academic setting in three related studies. Hall, McKay, and Mitsunaga (1971) explored the career patterns of deans of baccalaureate programs through a questionnaire survey. In a follow-up analysis, Mitsunaga and Hall (1976) used Gouldner's (1957, 1958) social identity theory to study manifest and latent identities of deans. The authors suggested that looking at latent identities may help to account for the success and happiness of some deans and the failure and dissatisfaction of others. Neither of the research reports was rigorous, and no overall profile of the dean was presented. In a third study, Hall, Mitsunaga, and deTornyay (1981) examined how a dean becomes interested in the position and what qualifications are necessary for it. Data from 99 women deans responding in 1970 were compared with data from 131 women deans responding in 1980. Results indicated that the contemporary dean is better prepared and has a greater interest in influencing the development of her school.

From a survey of "nurse influentials," Vance (1979) concluded that socialization and identity are two factors that influence advancement and success in female nurses as leaders. Because most of her sample had mentors and were mentors to others, she advocated the mentor system in nursing as a means of developing leadership. The report, however, only included the research in an incidental way to support her opinions; a complete summary of the study was not given.

Experimental designs were used in two studies in which the effects of educational programs on leadership development were investigated. The purpose of a study by Brock (1978) was to evaluate the impact of a management course on the leadership values, knowledge, and behaviors of senior baccalaureate nursing students. Results of this study demonstrated that an educational program could improve leadership knowledge and performance. In discussing her findings, Brock exhorted nurse educators to incorporate a management course into the curriculum for all students who are preparing to function as leaders. An earlier experimental study reported by Ingmire (1973) represented a substantial effort to document the effectiveness of a continuing education leadership program. Results of this multiphase study indicated that changes had occurred in the direction of the goals of the program.

In summary, most of the researchers who studied leadership development have described factors that may help identify, motivate, or socialize nurses into positions of leadership. Only two studies were found in which the effects of educational programs on leadership development were tested. Recommendations from these studies stressed the importance of identifying nurses with leadership potential early in their careers. Programs of continuing education, mentoring, and networking have been suggested as appropriate strategies for leadership development. These strategies needed further testing.

LEADERSHIP EFFECTIVENESS

Our review showed the largest number of studies to be in the category of leadership effectiveness. Therefore, the discussion is divided into two subcategories based on where the research was conducted, in the academic or practice setting. To distinguish this section from a previous one, the emphasis here is on evaluation of leadership effectiveness rather than on prediction of leadership success.

The Academic Setting

Research on leadership effectiveness in the academic setting has been of two types: studies of factors considered essential for effectiveness of deans, and studies of the effect of leadership on group performance. In the first group of studies leadership served as the dependent variable; in the second group leadership was manipulated as the independent variable.

In two studies (George, 1981; George & Deets, 1983) examined the effectiveness of deans in academic institutions. Assistant deans were described in the first study from the perspectives of career development, multiple roles, line or staff status, and role change recommendations. Few of the deans felt that they had adequate preparation for the job. The report was unclear as to sample selection, questionnaire development, and other details. A second study of deans had two purposes: to identify the perceived essential behaviors for functioning as a dean and to identify whether certain institutional and educational variables were related to dean behaviors. George and Deets concluded that although more deans today hold doctorates and have more continuing education opportunities available to them, few have new ideas about the dean's role. No reliability was reported for the questionnaire.

Deans' and others' perceptions of the dean's role were compared in two other studies (Higgs, 1978; Moloney, 1979). Higgs analyzed questionnaire responses from deans and faculty members to compare their perceptions of the degree to which the dean should and did participate in curriculum development. The questionnaire was pilot tested, with good reliability reported. In general, deans perceived themselves as being more involved than their faculty thought they were.

Moloney (1979) compared the leadership behavior of deans as perceived by the deans, their vice-presidents, and faculty. The Leadership Behavior Description Questionnaire (Stogdill, 1963) was used to obtain perceptions and expectations of the deans' leadership behavior. A 9-point rating scale for overall dean effectiveness was administered to vice-presidents and faculty. No reliability or validity measures were given for either instrument. Results showed that, in general, deans did not measure up to the expectations of either faculty or vice-presidents.

In a study with implications for leadership effectiveness in academia, Krampitz and Williams (1983) compared dean and faculty perceptions of the organizational climate in two baccalaureate programs. Four scales from Halpin and Croft's (1964) Organizational Climate Description Questionnaire were used to calculate a Climate Similarity Index. The authors concluded that the perceptions of faculty and deans differed, but they did not say how. The small sample size did not allow for generalizations.

Using leadership as the independent variable, one group of researchers studied the effect of leadership on group performance in a series of studies conducted in the late 1960s and early 1970s (McLaughlin, 1971; McLaughlin, Davis, & Reed, 1972; McLaughlin & White, 1973; McLaughlin, White, & Byfield, 1974). Subjects in all studies were nursing students taking group dynamics courses at the University of California. The methodology for the studies was quasi-experimental, with the experimental variables being leader time with the group, frequency and length of group meetings, use of programmed instruction, and use of videotape feedback. The study design improved with each investigation. Self-ratings of feelings and audiotapes of the group process were used as the performance measures. Although the findings were inconclusive, results showed that students preferred having the leader present, but that self-disclosure was better when the leader was not present.

In summary, most of the research concerned with leadership effectiveness in the academic setting has focused on the role of the dean. Even though mentoring and role modeling have been popular ideas with today's faculty, the effect of these variables on leadership performance has not been examined. Most of these studies were surveys of large samples. Statistics generally were limited to frequencies and chi-square tests. Often no reliability or validity was reported for the instruments. Several of the research reports were incomplete and confusing. Keeping in mind the methodological limitations, the research to date has suggested that the size of the organization and the nature of the faculty and educational programs may require different kinds of leadership expertise. The expectations of others have been important in determining leadership effectiveness. These findings were consistent with situational leadership theory. Research in this area showed that academic leaders could improve their performance and that better preparation for the leadership position was desirable.

The Practice Setting

One approach to studying leadership effectiveness in the practice setting has been to identify competencies of the leader. Like the research related to definition of leadership, these studies have added to the profile of characteristics, activities, and behaviors of leaders. They are discussed here, however, because of their focus on evaluation of the leaders' effectiveness. For example, the purpose of a large-scale investigation by Hagen and Wolff (1961) was to investigate the behaviors of head nurses, supervisors, and directors of nursing service that contributed to effective leadership. Eight hundred and twenty-four people in 15 hospitals were asked to describe incidents of effective and ineffective leadership behaviors. The extensive findings revealed that: (a) the roles of supervisor and head nurse in small hospitals were defined poorly, (b) directors were not perceived as providing leadership in long-range planning, (c) directors were perceived as ineffective in handling personnel, (d) the head nurse had the widest opportunities for leadership in regard to patient care, and (e) education did not predict leadership ability. This work, completed 25 years ago, still has merit for researchers and others currently interested in this area.

Although Hagen and Wolff questioned the overall competence of nurse administrators, it was not until much later that specific leadership competencies of nurse administrators were determined. Goodrich (1982) surveyed deans of accredited graduate programs and nursing directors of hospitals and home health agencies in a nine-state region in the South. Respondents were asked to rate the importance of and proficiency needed for 107 items grouped in the areas of nursing, leadership, organization, personnel management, resource management, security and safety, quality assurance, community, research, education, and trends. In both "importance" and "proficiency" areas, leadership was rated the highest. The same types and levels of competencies were needed by all administrators regardless of agency size, services provided, or staffing. Goodrich's study, like some others, was about perceptions of competence; it did not rate how people actually performed on the job.

Researchers have examined different groups to determine their perceptions of factors associated with leadership effectiveness. For example, in a study of staff nurses and nurse managers Goad and Moir (1981) found that perceptions of both groups of the ideal and actual nursing roles were congruent; leadership was included as a part of the ideal role. However, Bergman et al. (1981a, 1981b, 1981c) found that the perceptions of nurses, physicians, and administrators varied on what they considered to be desirable characteristics for head nurses. Head nurses disagreed with physicians and agency administrators on the importance of various activities, although they all agreed that head nurses should have physical and mental fitness, communication skills, clinical experience, variability of experience, continuity in nursing practice, and leadership abilities. In attempting to use their findings to reform the role of the head nurse in Israel, these authors may have reached certain conclusions about the need for reform before they began their investigation.

Basing a study on the proposition that nurse leaders exert a profound influence on nursing students, Smith (1965) compared the extent to which head nurses and nurse educators differed in their views about the desirable aspects of nursing practice. Head nurses were more concerned with appearance, conformity, friendliness, and cooperativeness. Educators valued emotional supportiveness, sensitivity, guidance, intelligence, and cognitive skills. Head nurses valued leadership more than educators did, and although both valued independence, neither valued the leadership characteristics of competition, directiveness, and determination. Smith inferred from the data that nursing students learn one set of expectations and then must perform with another. She recommended that schools of nursing strengthen the leadership training of students to prepare them to deal with conflicting values and expectations.

New graduates indeed have learned values from their teachers and experienced nurses. Bradley (1983) found that new graduates had a positive attitude toward leadership, although they equated leadership narrowly with a team management position. One implication would be that schools of nursing should provide broader leadership definition and experiences for students.

Differing expectations were also the subject of a study by Anderson (1964a, 1964b). Her findings showed that supervisors preferred head nurses who liked coordinating activities and that subordinates preferred head nurses who liked nursing care activities. Differing expectations of others made the role of head nurse more difficult.

Ludemann (1983) studied the congruence between management style and organizational needs by surveying subordinates, directors of nursing, and hospital administrators in 500 randomly selected hospitals. Her findings indicated that many hospital and nursing leaders experienced a lack of congruence between their leadership style and the style indicated by the developmental stage of the organization. The implication of this study was a need to match the leadership style of the manager with the needs of the organization. In order to be effective managers must recognize their own preferred leadership styles and adapt those styles to meet the needs of the organization.

In a rare longitudinal study, Baker (1979) followed 50 nurses from 50 hospitals over 5 years to ascertain the differences in life goal patterns of successful and unsuccessful nursing leaders. A successful nurse was promoted to at least a head nurse position within 1 year of the initial testing, was still in at least a head nurse position 5 years later, and was ranked by the director of nursing in the top third of nurses based on leadership ability. Successful nurses had a different pattern of life goals than unsuccessful nurses. Life goals that elicited the greatest differences between these two groups were self-expression, independence, leadership, and security. Findings indicated that the unsuccessful nurses were unwilling or unable to change their life goals, whereas the successful nurses' life goals became more congruent with the leadership role itself. Based on these results, Baker recommended that educational programs be developed to help the nurse who is interested in a leadership role build life goals that are consistent with that role.

Although a number of investigators have implied that education was a key to leadership effectiveness, this relationship was investigated in only two studies. In both studies, leadership was included as part of a measure of job performance. In a national survey Dyer, Cope, Monson, and Van Drimmelen (1972) sampled 1,018 nurses from 31 VA hospitals and compared their self-ratings on several scales with the ratings by their supervisors. Nurses who scored high on leadership surpassed 90% of their class academically, worked as instructors and supervisors for a period of 3 to 6 years, presented papers and published articles, had opportunities for creative expression, and worked independently and diligently to obtain their goals. In another study, McCloskey (1983a, 1983b) investigated whether nurses with different educational preparation differed in job effectiveness; leadership was measured as one aspect. Self-ratings and head nurse ratings were obtained from a sample of 299 staff nurses from 12 randomly selected hospitals in the Chicago area. Leadership skills were rated lower by head nurses than by the nurses themselves. No difference was found for leadership skills of associate degree, diploma, and baccalaureate nurses, although all three groups had better leadership skills than practical nurses.

Much of the research on leadership effectiveness has focused on the effect of leadership on the followers, or subordinates, within an organization. To illustrate, the purpose of a descriptive study by White (1971a, 1971b) was to obtain perceptions of nurses regarding the attitudes and behaviors of effective and weak managers. Head nurses and supervisory nurses were asked to rate known effective and ineffective managers. Effective managers were more likely to use subordinates' ideas and knowledge, were more sensitive to their problems, shared information, exhibited trust and confidence, and gave rewards and guidance. Overall, effective managers had a more participative style. White (1971b) concluded that the behavior of subordinates of effective managers was more positive because the leadership style of the effective managers was more appropriate. Although this investigator measured beliefs rather than actual performance, it demonstrated that subordinates could distinguish between effective and ineffective leaders.

One investigator, using an experimental approach, measured the effects of leadership behavior on subordinate performance. In a well-designed study, Stull (1983) examined the effects of supervisor feedback and goal setting on staff nurse performance. Head nurses and staff nurses from one VA hospital in the Midwest were assigned to four experimental groups and one control group. Treatments were assigned randomly. Staff nurse performance was measured by the

Schwirian Scale (1979). Unfortunately, the research report was focused on a lengthy literature review and methodological considerations; results of the study were not included.

Retention and job satisfaction also were outcomes of leadership effectiveness. Shoemaker and El-Ahraf (1983) concluded that decentralization of decision making led to increased job satisfaction and decreased turnover. Twenty hospitals in California participated in the research, but the sample was not described adequately in the report. However, the article was more a testimonial to the benefits of decentralization than a summary of research findings. Nealey and Blood (1968) studied the relationships of leader style and leader behavior to work-group performance and subordinate job satisfaction. Head nurses and supervisors were rated by subordinates. Head nurses who were task-oriented received higher performance ratings, whereas supervisors who were more considerate received higher ratings. Subordinates' job satisfaction was related positively to both head nurse and supervisor consideration. The authors concluded that the findings pointed to differences in situational leadership demands at different organizational levels.

Pryer and Distefano (1971) found that when attendants, aides, and nurses working in a state mental hospital perceived their supervisors as considerate they were more satisfied. Aides' satisfaction also was correlated with their perception of the supervisor as providing structure. Unfortunately, many variables that could have affected job satisfaction were not controlled in this study.

Using a sample of staff nurses in neonatal intensive care units, Duxbury, Armstrong, Drew, and Henly (1984) also found a positive relationship between head nurse consideration and staff nurse satisfaction. Analysis of the data indicated that low consideration and high structure of head nurses were associated with low satisfaction and burnout of their staff nurses.

In summary, leadership effectiveness in nursing practice has been the subject of numerous research efforts. Leadership effectiveness has been determined by identifying specific competencies of the leader, by examining congruency of role expectations and behaviors, and by studying factors that influenced leadership effectiveness. Leadership effectiveness has been measured by retention in the leadership position over time and by job performance and satisfaction of the followers.

Researchers of leadership effectiveness in nursing practice have identified directors, supervisors, and head nurses as leaders. Some have looked at the leadership qualities of staff nurses. Like the research on academic administrators, the studies of leadership in the practice setting were mostly descriptive in nature, and many focused on perceptions of the leadership role. The quality of the reports was somewhat better than those on academic leadership; the methodologies and theoretical frameworks were more diverse. The terms leadership and management often were used interchangeably in the nursing practice literature. Certain behaviors by deans were called leadership, whereas the same behaviors by directors of nursing service or head nurses were referred to as management. In at least two studies the importance of decision-making skills was demonstrated. Although role preparation of nurse executives has improved in recent years, better preparation still is necessary. Authors, however, were not specific about what comprised better leadership training.

CONCLUSIONS AND RECOMMENDATIONS FOR FUTURE RESEARCH

As this review began we were uncertain about whether there was sufficient research on leadership nursing to comprise a substantive area of study. The 58 research reports that were found constituted a good beginning effort to define and describe systematically the characteristics of leadership. In categorizing these research efforts, one could see that the majority of studies fell into two areas: defining leadership and leadership effectiveness in the practice setting. This suggested that nurses have been concerned most with developing a conception of leadership and with understanding its impact within an organizational context.

The research reports were found in a variety of nursing journals. However, most of them were published in three journals: *Nursing Research, Nursing Leadership*, and *Nursing Outlook*. Some of the reports were published in a book or monograph form. Although a substantial number of the researchers investigated leadership effectiveness in the practice setting, only two studies were reported in journals frequently read by administrators. Most studies published in the research journals included specific details of the research methodology and analysis of data, but the reports often were unwieldy in length and dull to read. Conversely, the research reports published in other journals were usually interesting to read, but salient information about the research design and methodology often was missing.

Measurement of leadership was a problem because there still has been little agreement about the meaning of this concept. In addressing this problem, an early approach was to define leadership through case study and group profiles. Another approach has been to develop instruments that measured leadership attributes or behaviors and then to use these instruments to predict leadership or evaluate its effectiveness. It was apparent that any systematic study of leadership in nursing would depend on valid and reliable measurement of the concept. To expedite future research efforts, the instruments that have been developed are summarized in Table 8-1. Some of these tools have been developed by social psychologists and organizational theorists; others have been designed by nurses. Some of these instruments also are found in *The Experience of Work: A Compendium and Review of 249 Measures and Their Uses* (Cook, Hepworth, Wall, & Warr, 1981).

Examination of Table 8-1 will show that the Leader Behavior Description Questionnaire (LBDQ) (Stodgill, 1963; Stogdill & Coons, 1957) is the oldest and best-known measure of leadership, and was used in five of the research reports that we reviewed. Although none of the investigators used the Situational Leadership Instruments (Greene, 1980; Hersey and Blanchard, 1982), they have been included because they are of recent origin and are some of the best tools currently available. The majority of instruments listed in the table have been developed for use in fields other than nursing. The instruments developed for nursing tend to measure leadership as one aspect of job performance. Some of the instruments measure leadership style, while others measure specific leadership behaviors, and still others measure values and opinions about leadership. Some have well-established validity and reliability; others, however, still need further validation or reliability testing. Despite these limitations, future investigators of leadership in nursing should consider use of these instruments in preference to the development of new measures.

Most researchers have used a survey approach to study leadership; many of them have elicited perceptions of leadership rather than actual leadership performance. Sufficient evidence is available from these descriptive studies to move toward research methodologies that include correlation or predictive analysis. Although longitudinal stud-

Table 8-1   Instruments to Measure Leadership

Instrument and Author(s)	Description	Studies in Which Instrument Was Used
1. Leader Behavior Description Questionnaire (Stodgill & Coons, 1957; Stogdill, 1963)	Oldest, best known, and most often used measure of leadership. Covers 12 aspects of leadership measuring behavior through descriptions from followers. Most frequently used scales are Initiating Structure and Consideration. Reliability of .87 for Consideration (police officers) and .80 for Initiating Structure (college presidents). Items differ by study, and investigators did not report new reliabilities. See Cook, Hepworth, Wall, and Warr, 1981.	Anderson, 1964a, 1964b; Moloney, 1979; Pryer & Distefano, 1971; Nealey & Blood, 1968; Sheridan & Vredenburgh, 1978
2. Least Preferred Co-worker (Fiedler, 1967; Fiedler, Mahar, & Chemars, 1977)	Individual describes person most difficult to work with. Based on attitudes toward this person, individual is classified as relationship oriented or task oriented. Much discussion in the literature as to what the scale really measures. Split half reliability, .90. See Cook, Hepworth, Wall, & Warr, 1981.	Nealey & Blood, 1968
3. Situational Leadership Instruments: a. Lead-Self b. Lead-Other c. Power-Perception— Profile, Self, and Other (Greene, 1980; Hersey & Blanchard, 1982)	Collection of rating scales to determine leadership style or power as perceived by self and others. Scoring results in a style profile. Lead-Self was standardized through the responses of 264 North American managers. Reliability and validity estimates on Lead-Self available in Greene (1980); none reported for Lead-Other and Power-Perception Profile.	

Table 8-1 *Continued*

Instrument and Author(s)	Description	Studies in Which Instrument Was Used
4. Leadership Value Scale (Gordon, 1975)	Assesses a person's value of leadership. Consists of 16 sets of three statements from Gordon's Survey of Interpersonal Values. For each item respondent indicates what is most important and what is least important. Test-retest reliability coefficient, $r = .88$; K-R reliability, .83.	Brock, 1978
5. Leadership Opinion Questionnaire (Fleishman, 1969)	Measures leaders' opinions about desirable leadership behavior. Two 20-item scales to be self-administered to measure leadership consideration and structure; reliabilities (alpha) of .91 for consideration and .78 for structure reported by Duxbury et al., 1984. See Cook, Hepworth, Wall, and Warr, 1981.	Duxbury, Armstrong, Drew, & Henly, 1984.
6. Managerial Key for The California Psychological Inventory (Gough, 1969; Goodstein & Schraeder, 1963)	Contains 206 items to measure 18 personality traits associated with effective management/leadership, including dominance, aggressiveness, ambition, self-confidence, and flexibility. Validated in 1963 by comparing top-rated managers with those not so rated.	Gilbert, 1975
7. Schwirian Six-Dimension Scale of Nursing Performance (Schwirian, 1979)	A 52-item, 6-factor scale to measure performance of nurses; Leadership subscale has five items. Well constructed with good validity and reliability. See McCloskey, 1983.	McCloskey, 1983a, 1983b; Schwirian, 1979; Stull, 1983

(continued)

Table 8-1 *Continued*

Instrument and Author(s)	Description	Studies in Which Instrument Was Used
8. Competencies needed by Nurse Administrators (Goodrich, 1982)	A 117-item questionnaire to identify type and level of competencies needed by nurse administrators in the following areas: nursing, leadership, organization, personnel management, resource management, security and safety, quality assurance, community, research, education, trends. Leadership area has 16 items. Good validity. Reliability ascertained by correlating mean of each item with total scale mean.	Goodrich, 1982
9. Head Nurse Behavior Description Scales (HNBDS), Nurse Performance Description Scales (NPDS), and Descriptive Scales for Nursing Performance (DSNP) (Dyer, Cope, Monson, & Van Drimmelen, 1972)	HNBDS Assesses the psychological atmosphere of the ward. Consists of 45 questions in 4 subscales: consideration, aloofness, thrust, and production emphasis. No reliability or validity reported. NPDS and DSNP assess nurse performance. NPDS has 5 subscales: professional orientation, thrust, consideration, clinical competence, leading, and teaching. DSNP has 16 subscales including group leadership and leadership adroitness. Reported validities range from .40 to .70 and reliabilities mostly in high .80s.	Dyer, Cope, Monson, & Van Drimmelen, 1972
10. Dean Effectiveness Scale (Seeman, 1960; Moloney, 1979)	Measures overall leadership effectiveness of deans. Nine items rated on a scale of 1 to 5. No reliability or validity reported.	Moloney, 1979

ies are costly and time consuming, they would be particularly useful in evaluating the effect of leadership development programs on leadership success. Although continuing education, mentoring, and networking have been proposed as methods of leadership development, virtually no researchers have tested these methods. More research is needed with leadership introduced as the independent variable so that its effect on the organization and human relation can be determined. There has been a trend toward analyzing leadership effectiveness according to job performance and satisfaction of subordinates. However, most of this research has been conducted in acute care rather than community or academic settings.

The results of the review suggest that leadership effectiveness is related largely to situational variables. A match between situational variables and personality attributes or management style appears to be a key in preventing role conflict and in fostering effective job performance and subordinate satisfaction. More research would help to document the congruency of factors associated with leadership effectiveness. Investigators who have used personality and interest inventories indicate that certain attributes and interests can be used to predict leadership potential. This evidence could be used as a basis for targeting persons to participate in leadership development activities. Longitudinal studies where potential leaders are followed through programs of continuing education, or through mentoring or networking experiences, into positions of leadership in complex organizations could yield some useful information.

Although the findings in nursing that suggest that leadership effectiveness is related to the situation are consistent with general leadership theory, the role of nurse leader is made particularly difficult by the changing health care scene. There is no doubt that the concept of leadership in nursing is more complex today than 20 years ago. Nursing leaders are in positions of responsibility associated with policy formation and decision making in complex organizations. Many of these nurses still are not prepared adequately for their responsibilities. There is some research to document a positive relationship between educational preparation and leadership effectiveness, but what that educational preparation should be is not clear. Because there is an association between management style and situational factors, the need for educational preparation and personality variables may vary from one organization to another and within the same organization over time. Thus, the key is to develop appropriate knowledge and skill and then to be astute and flexible in adapting to situational needs. This poses a great challenge to contemporary nursing leaders because of the rapid changes that have occurred within the profession and in health care delivery.

Research has yielded some evidence to help us in accepting this challenge. Leadership effectiveness, regardless of the situation, requires skill in the areas of decision making, communication, interpersonal relationships, conflict management, change, and risk taking. In applying these skills it is important to assess the expectations of both superiors and subordinates and the needs of the organization to achieve role congruency. Studies have shown that, in general, a participative style and consideration tend to be more effective in most nursing situations than an authoritarian style and overreliance on structure. The personality traits of warmth and assertiveness and a positive view of self and others also have been associated with leadership effectiveness.

Further research is recommended in the following areas: the effects of different types of leadership on the satisfaction and performance of subordinates, further study of situational variables and role expectations on leadership effectiveness, experimental and longitudinal analysis of the effect of leadership development strategies on leadership success, comparison studies of leaders in multiple settings, and further testing of the instruments developed to measure leadership performance. Multivariate designs should be used to analyze leader performance.

The research on nursing leadership has demonstrated that this is a substantive area worthy of study. That we face a leadership crisis in nursing has been reported in the professional literature. The researchers whose work is reviewed in this chapter have delineated the parameters of need. Aggressive research in the coming decade will help us face the challenge.

REFERENCES

Anderson, R. M. (1964a). Activity preferences and leadership behavior of head nurses: Part 1. *Nursing Research, 13*, 239–243.

Anderson, R. M. (1964b). Activity preferences and leadership behavior of head nurses: Part 2. *Nursing Research, 13*, 333–337.

Aydelotte, M. K. (1984). *Report of the 1982 survey of nursing service administrators*. Chicago: American Hospital Association and American Society for

Nurse Administrators.

Baker, C. M. (1981). Leadership behaviors of academic middle managers in nursing. In S. Ketefian (Ed.), *Perspectives on nursing leadership* (pp. 11-25). New York: Teachers College Press.

Baker, W. G. III. (1979). Changes in life goals as related to success in a nursing leadership role. *Nursing Research, 28*, 234-236.

Bergman, R., Stockler, R. A., Shavit, N., Sharon, R., Feinberg, D., & Danon, A. (1981a). Role, selection and preparation of unit head nurses – I. *International Journal of Nursing Studies, 18*, 123-152.

Bergman, R., Stockler, R. A., Shavit, N., Sharon, R., Feinberg, D., & Danon, A. (1981b). Role, selection and preparation of unit head nurses – II. *International Journal of Nursing Studies, 18*, 191-211.

Bergman, R., Stockler, R. A., Shavit, N., Sharon, R., Feinberg, D., & Danon, A. (1981c). Role, selection and preparation of unit head nurses – III. *International Journal of Nursing Studies, 18*, 237-250.

Bradley, J. C. (1983). Nurses' attitudes toward dimensions of nursing practice. *Nursing Research, 32*, 110-114.

Brimmer, P. F., Skoner, M. M., Pender, N. S., Williams, C. A., Lleming, J. W., & Werley, H. H. (1983). Nurses with doctoral degrees: Education and employment characteristics. *Research in Nursing and Health, 6*, 157-165.

Brock, A. M. (1978). Impact of a management oriented course on knowledge and leadership skills exhibited by baccalaureate nursing students. *Nursing Research, 27*, 217-221.

Campbell, D. P. (1977). *Manual for the SVIB-SCII* (2nd ed.). Stanford, CA: Stanford University Press.

Cattell, R. B., Eber, H. W., & Tatsuoka, M. M. (1974). *Handbook for the 16 Personality Factor Questionnaire*. Champaign, IL: Institute for Personality and Ability Testing.

Christy, T. E. (1969a). Portrait of a leader: M. Adelaide Nutting. *Nursing Outlook, 17*(1), 20-24.

Christy, T. E. (1969b). Portrait of a leader: Isabel Hampton Robb. *Nursing Outlook, 17*(3), 26-29.

Christy, T. E. (1969c). Portrait of a leader: Lavinia Lloyd Dock. *Nursing Outlook, 17*(6), 72-75.

Christy, T. E. (1969d). Portrait of a leader: Isabel Maitland Stewart. *Nursing Outlook, 17*(10), 44-48.

Christy, T. E. (1970a). Portrait of a leader: Lillian D. Wald. *Nursing Outlook, 18*(3), 50-54.

Christy, T. E. (1970b). Portrait of a leader: Annie Warbuton Goodrich. *Nursing Outlook, 18*(8), 46-50.

Christy, T. E. (1975). Portrait of a leader: Sophia F. Palmer. *Nursing Outlook, 23*, 746-751.

Cook, J. D., Hepworth, S. J., Wall, T. D., & Warr, P. B. (1981). *The experience of work: A compendium and review of 249 measures and their uses*. New York: Academic Press.

Corona, D. (1981). Who's who among nursing leaders. *Nursing Leadership, 4*(2), 5-11.

Davidson, L. C. (1968). Students' perception of leadership in nursing care. *Nursing Outlook, 16*(12), 30-31.

Demi, A. S., & Miles, M. S. (1984). An examination of nursing leadership following a disaster. *Topics in Clinical Nursing, 6*, 63-78.

Duxbury, M. L., Armstrong, G. D., Drew, D. J., & Henly, S. J. (1984). Head nurse leadership style with staff nurse burnout and job satisfaction in neonatal intensive care units. *Nursing Research, 33*, 97–101.

Dyer, E. D., Cope, M. J., Monson, M. A., & Van Drimmelen, J. B. (1972). Can job performance be predicted from biographical, personality and administrative climate inventories? *Nursing Research, 21*, 294–304.

Fiedler, F. E. (1967). *A theory of leadership effectiveness.* New York: McGraw-Hill.

Fiedler, F. E., Mahar, L., & Chemars, M. M. (1977). *Leadership match IV: Programmed instruction in leadership in the U.S. Army.* Alexandria, VA: U.S. Army Research Institute.

Fleishman, E. A. (1969). *Manual for leader opinion questionnaire.* Chicago: Science Research Associates.

Friss, L. (1983). Organization commitment and job involvement of directors of nursing services. *Nursing Administration Quarterly, 7*(2), 1–18.

George, S. A. (1981). Associate and assistant deanships in schools of nursing. *Nursing Leadership, 4*(3), 25–30.

George, S. A., & Deets, C. (1983). Top academic nurse administrators' perceptions of essential behaviors for their positions. *Nursing Leadership, 6*(2), 44–55.

George, V. D. (1982). Profile: Black deans of nursing programs. *Nursing Leadership, 5*(4), 23–29.

Gilbert, M. A. (1975). Personality profiles and leadership potential of medical-surgical and psychiatric nursing graduate students. *Nursing Research, 24*, 125–130.

Gluck, M., & Charter, R. (1980). Personal qualities of nurses implying need for continuing education to increase interpersonal and leadership effectiveness. *The Journal of Continuing Education in Nursing, 11*(4), 29–36.

Goad, S., & Moir, G. (1981). Role discrepancy: Implications for nursing leaders. *Nursing Leadership, 4*(2), 23–27.

Goodrich, N. M. (1982). *A profile of the competent nursing administrator.* Ann Arbor: UMI Research Press.

Goodstein, L. D., & Schraeder, N. J. (1963). An empirically derived managerial key for the California Psychological Inventory. *Journal of Applied Psychology, 47*, 42–45.

Gordon, L. V. (1975). *Survey of interpersonal values manual.* Chicago: Science Research Associates.

Gough, H. G. (1969). *Manual for the California Psychological Inventory* (rev. ed.). Palo Alto, CA: Consulting Psychologists Press.

Gouldner, A. W. (1957). Cosmopolitans and locals: Toward an analysis of latent social roles—I. *Administrative Science Quarterly, 2*(3), 281–306.

Gouldner, A. W. (1958). Cosmopolitans and locals: Toward an analysis of latent social roles—II. *Administrative Science Quarterly, 2*(4), 444–480.

Greene, J. F. (1980). *A summary of technical information about lead-self.* San Diego, CA: University Associates.

Hagen, E., & Wolff, L. (1961). *Nursing leadership behavior in general hospitals.* New York: Teachers College, Columbia University, Institute of Research and Service in Nursing Education.

Hall, B. A., McKay, R. D., & Mitsunaga, B. K. (1971). Dimensions of role commitment: Career patterns of deans of nursing. In M. V. Batey (Ed.), *Communicating Nursing Research: Vol. 5. Is the Gap Being Bridged?* (pp.

84–106). Boulder, CO: Western Interstate Commission for Higher Education.

Hall, B. A., Mitsunaga, G. K., & deTornyay, R. (1981). Deans of nursing: Changing socialization patterns. *Nursing Outlook, 29*, 92–95.

Halpin, A. W., & Croft, D. R. (1964). Organizational climate of schools: A research paper. Chicago: University of Chicago, Midwest Administration Center.

Hanson, H. A., & Chater, S. (1983). Role selection by nurses: Managerial interests and personal attributes. *Nursing Research, 32*, 48–52.

Hersey, P., & Blanchard, K. W. (1982). *Management of organizational behavior: Utilizing human resources* (4th ed.). Englewood Cliffs, NJ: Prentice-Hall.

Higgs, Z. R. (1978). Expectations and perceptions of the curricular leadership role of administrators of nursing education units. *Nursing Research, 27*, 57–63.

Holland, J. L. (1978). *Manual for the Vocational Preference Inventory*. Palo Alto, CA: Consulting Psychologists Press.

Ingmire, A. E. (1973). The effectiveness of a leadership programme in nursing. *International Journal of Nursing Studies, 10*, 3–19.

Johnson, B. M. (1983). *The dean of nursing: A descriptive survey with comparisons between nursing and social work deans*. Washington, DC: American Association of Colleges of Nursing.

Jones, N. K., & Jones, J. W. (1979). The head nurse: A managerial definition of the activity role set. *Nursing Administration Quarterly, 3*(2), 45–57.

Kelly, W. L. (1974). Psychological predictions of leadership in nursing. *Nursing Research, 23*, 38–42.

Knudson, E. G. (1968). Public health nurses' interests in occupational advancement. *Nursing Research, 17*, 327–335.

Krampitz, S. D., & Williams, M. (1983). Organizational climate: A measure of faculty and nurse administrator perception. *Journal of Nursing Education, 22*, 200–206.

Langford, T. (1983). Who's who among nursing leaders. *Nursing Leadership, 6*(2), 61–66.

Ludemann, R. (1983). Fit or misfit: A comparison of hospital and nursing managers' perceptions of their roles and their organizations. In B. Mark (Ed.), *Proceedings of the Second National Conference on Nursing Administration Research* (pp. 220–239). Richmond, VA: Virginia Commonwealth University.

McCloskey, J. C. (1983a). Nursing education and job effectiveness. *Nursing Research, 32*, 53–58.

McCloskey, J. C. (1983b). *Toward an educational model of nursing effectiveness*. Ann Arbor, MI: UMI Research Press.

McLaughlin, F. E. (1971). Personality changes through alternate group leadership. *Nursing Research, 20*, 123–130.

McLaughlin, F. E., Davis, M. L., & Reed, S. L. (1972). Effects of three types of group leadership structures on the self-perceptions of undergraduate nursing students. *Nursing Research, 21*, 244–257.

McLaughlin, F. E., & White, E. (1973). Small group functioning under six different leadership formats. *Nursing Research, 22*, 37–54.

McLaughlin, F. E., White, E., & Byfield, B. (1974). Modes of interpersonal feedback and leadership structure in six small groups. *Nursing Research, 23*, 307–318.

Mitsunaga, B. K., & Hall, B. A. (1976). The deanship: Manifest and latent identity. *Nursing Outlook, 24*, 292–296.

Moloney, M. M. (1979). *Leadership in nursing: Theory, strategies, action* (pp. 140–149). St. Louis: Mosby.

Nealey, S. M., & Blood, M. R. (1968). Leadership performance of nursing supervisors at two organizational levels. *Journal of Applied Psychology, 52*, 414–422.

Pryer, M. W., & Distefano, M. K. (1971). Perceptions of leadership behavior, job satisfaction and internal–external control across three nursing levels. *Nursing Research, 20*, 534–537.

Reddin, W. J. (1970). *Managerial effectiveness.* New York: McGraw-Hill.

Schwirian, P. M. (1977). Prediction of successful nursing performance (Parts I and II, Publication No. HRA 77-27). Washington, DC: Department of Health, Education, and Welfare.

Schwirian, P. M. (1978). Evaluating the performance of nurses: A multi-dimensional approach. *Nursing Research, 27*, 347–351.

Schwirian, P. M. (1979). Prediction of successful nursing performance (Parts III and IV, Publication No. HRA 79-15). Washington, DC: Department of Health, Education, and Welfare.

Seeman, M. (1960). *Social status and leadership.* Columbus, OH: Ohio State University. Bureau of Educational Research and Service.

Sheridan, J. E., & Vredenburgh, D. J. (1978). Predicting leadership behavior in a hospital organization. *Academy of Management Journal, 21*, 679–689.

Shoemaker, H., & El-Ahraf, A. (1983). Decentralization of nursing service management and its impact on job satisfaction. *Nursing Administration Quarterly, 7*(2), 69–76.

Sills, G. M. (1978). Hildegard E. Peplau: Leader, practitioner, academician, scholar and theorist. *Perspectives in Psychiatric Care, 16*, 122–128.

Smith, K. M. (1965). Discrepancies in the role-specific values of head nurses and nursing educators. *Nursing Research, 14*, 196–202.

Stogdill, R. M. (1963). *Manual for the leader behavior description questionnaire—Form XII: An experimental revision.* Columbus, OH: Ohio State University, Bureau of Business Research.

Stogdill, R. M., & Coons, A. E. (1957). *Leader behavior: Its description and measurement* (Ohio Studies in Personnel: Research Monograph No. 88). Columbus, OH: Ohio State University, Bureau of Business Research.

Stull, M. K. (1983). Improving the performance of staff nurses through goal-setting and performance feedback: Theoretical and methodological considerations. In B. Mark (Ed.), *Proceedings of the Second National Conference on Nursing Administration Research* (pp. 307–341). Richmond, VA: Virginia Commonwealth University.

Survey of perceived relationships between chief operating officers and directors of nurses. (1977). *Hospital Topics, 55*(2), 38–40.

Vance, C. N. (1979). Women leaders: Modern day heroines or societal deviants? *Image: The Journal of Nursing Scholarship, 11*(2), 37–41.

White, H. C. (1971a). Perceptions of leadership styles of nurses in supervisory positions. *Journal of Nursing Administration, 1*(2), 44–51.

White, H. C. (1971b). Some perceived behavior and attitudes of hospital employees under effective and ineffective supervisors. *Journal of Nursing Administration, 1*(1), 49–54.

PART V

Other Research

Chapter 9

International Nursing Research

AFAF IBRAHIM MELEIS
SCHOOL OF NURSING
UNIVERSITY OF CALIFORNIA, SAN FRANCISCO

CONTENTS

The reviews and recommendations of Margretta Styles, Susan Gortner, and anonymous
reviewers are greatly appreciated. Help and assistance in reviewing, locating, and organizing
the literature for the analysis was provided by Diana Canto, Ardis Hanson, Nancy Hardies,
Dawn Hasegawa, Sharon Hooey, Chuck Marion, Chuck Pitkofsky, Hanna Regev, Sandra
Rogers, Patricia Seabrooks, Torrey Stadtner, Tamara Ward, Margaret Warrick, and Victoria
Weaver. The author also acknowledges the editorial assistance of Erika Hublitz.

International research in nursing contributes to the development of nursing knowledge. At present, international research still requires delineation and definition that can be achieved best by a thorough review of the literature. In this chapter, the state of the art of international nursing research is reviewed, based on reported research. A proposed role for international research is related to nursing through the identification of trends and future directions. Recommendations are presented on ways nurses can use international work to enhance research, and how nurse researchers can participate in developing and expanding international studies. The conceptual schema used in organizing the research findings evolved from an extensive review of literature in nursing and other fields.

DEFINITION

International nursing research represents comparative research on nursing phenomena conducted in more than one country. A more specific definition of international nursing research would be as follows:

1. Research conducted cross-nationally to test propositions or theories.
2. Research of subject matter other than that generated in the United States.
3. Research reported in the United States or internationally that included subjects who resided outside the United States.
4. Research by foreign nurses in their countries reported in an international or U.S. journal.
5. Research by a foreign nurse in the United States who uses a U.S. or foreign sample.

Review and critique of international research should also include multinational as well as national research. The above definition accounts for the present status of nursing research and is based on the premise that nursing knowledge can progress if its propositions are examined in culturally diverse samples. The definition of international nursing research that was used as a guide for the present review and critique includes research representative of global nursing phenomena published in the United States or in international nursing journals.

PROCESS OF REVIEW

International nursing research usually has spanned several disciplines, such as public health, international relations, political science, sociology, anthropology, and psychology. Nurse investigators frequently have explored questions that have implications for knowledge development in areas other than nursing. For the purpose of this report it was, however, necessary to confine this review to nursing sources. All nursing indexes published through September 1984 were reviewed for articles related to cross-national research, research based outside the United States, and international nursing in general. Using the key words *international, cross-cultural, immigration, foreign,* and *nursing,* a MEDLINE search was conducted for articles that fell within the definition. A second MEDLINE search was done for abstracts with the above key words. A key journal in which nursing research has been published in the fields of social science and medicine also was included (Bryant, 1980; Kleczkowski, 1980; Meleis, 1979c, 1982b). All quantitative and a small number of qualitative articles that met the criteria were selected from the searches and issue-by-issue review of *Cancer Nursing, International Journal of Nursing Studies, International Nursing Review, Journal of Advanced Nursing, Nursing Research, Research in Nursing and Health,* and *Western Journal of Nursing Research.* The inclusive dates of the journals that were reviewed were 1960 to 1984. *International Journal of Nursing Studies* issues preceding 1971 were not available, and the review of that journal was from 1971 to 1984.

AREAS OF INVESTIGATION IN
INTERNATIONAL RESEARCH

Manpower Analyses and Investigations

Shortages of nurses and shortages in nursing care of patients have been issues in many countries. It was not surprising that international nurse investigators were concerned with the values associated with choosing nursing as a career, choosing the type of educational programs, the problems of attrition and retention in nursing education and practice, and the varied perceptions of the role, image, and status of nursing. Patterns of choice and commitments to nursing were explored by investigators in many countries. For students tested during the first and third years in four Swedish schools of nursing, the findings pointed to a decreased pattern of future commitment to nursing that was associated with an increase in their authoritarianism (Adler, 1969). The American scientists Croog, Caudill, and Blumen (1968) studied nursing students at two religious institutions in Japan. Christian-oriented Japanese students indicated that they selected nursing for altruistic and ideal reasons such as the desire to serve humanity; students from traditional Oriental religions indicated pragmatic reasons for their occupational selection, such as economic security and developing the highest level of professional skills.

The image and status of a nurse were variables related to recruitment and retention of nurses. In a 10-year study of northern European countries, Kruse and Munck (1965) concluded that the community image and status of nurses were more significant variables in negotiations over salary and employment conditions than such variables as type of work, level of responsibility, and education. The image and status of nursing also have been identified by nurses as significant variables promoting nurses' emigration from developing countries to more developed countries (Ronaghy, Zeighami, Agah, Rouhani, & Zimmer, 1975).

Another group of studies was centered on types of, and resources for, nursing education (Bergman, Krulik, & Ditzian, 1976; de Castro, Lunardi, Coloriti, & de Moura, 1976; Henkle, 1979; Jato, Mounlom, Colgate, & Carrière, 1979; Kruse & Munck, 1965). Perceptions of the role of the nurse as seen by nurses (de Castro, Lunardi, Coloriti, & de Moura, 1976; Jaeger-Burns, 1981; Kelly, 1973), by institutions (Baudry, 1978), and by social workers (Bergman, Krulik, & Ditzian, 1976) support the varied patterns of perceptions that were demonstrated in the United States. The authors of this group of studies utilized descriptive, phenomenological existential, or ethnographic studies. Some were based on samples from one nation. When comparative designs were used, few investigators used cross-national samples (Beck, 1965; Bhanumathi, 1977; Henkle, 1979; Jaeger-Burns, 1981). Other investigators effectively used countries in the same geographical region in their comparisons (Jato, Mounlom, Colgate, & Carrière, 1979; Kruse & Munck, 1965).

Immigration of Nurses

In a country of limited resources, the "brain drain" of emigrating nurses is particularly taxing on patient care, whereas in a country with ample resources, immigrating professionals may have caused an abundance of the overqualified (Logan, 1980). This concern was reflected in the findings of a multinational study on the migration of nurses and physicians by the World Health Organization (WHO) (Mejia, Pizurki, & Royston, 1979). The investigators used data provided by member countries of the International Council of Nurses (ICN). Some 15,000 nurses left their country of origin or training yearly, representing a migration of 0.5% of the nurses of the world, a figure almost equal to the 0.6% of physicians of the world who emigrated. Researchers who focused on emigration from a specific country, such as India (Bachu, 1973) or Iran (Ronaghy et al., 1975), indicated that nurses emigrate because of (a) limited resources in their own country, (b) a preference for urban over rural employment, (c) a preference for working conditions found in developed countries, and (d) a perceived difference in the image and status of nurses in the host country over their own country.

The WHO (1979) study represented a model of the multiplicity of data sources needed in cross-national research. The various types of data came from censuses, professional registries, licensing authorities, and migration data bases. Reliability of the data was, however, limited because of variability in the accuracy of reporting and recording. Reliability of data in international studies could be enhanced by using multiple sources.

Primary Care Nursing

Primary care nursing is of great importance because it was named by WHO and the United Nations Childrens' Emergency Fund (WHO/ UNICEF, 1978) as the mechanism through which health for all could be achieved. The concepts *primary nursing* and *primary health care nursing* frequently are used interchangeably. Primary nursing may be viewed as a supervention of professional nursing practice (Hegyvary, 1982); primary health care nursing supervenes, enlarges, or encompasses community health care nursing (Collière, 1980; Jaeger-Burns, 1981). Shared elements in both types of nursing are comprehensiveness of care, collaboration in care, active participation of nurse and client or client group, emphasis on care that takes into account curative measures, enjoyment of a good degree of autonomy on the part of the nurse, integration of the social dimension, a total view and analysis of the situation by the nurse, and accountability of the nurse for the care provided. The differences are in the personnel and setting. Primary nursing is practiced by nurses within the confines of the hospital, whereas primary health care nursing is practiced in the community by nurses and community workers. The latter stresses the nurse's role in primary health care in general. Primary health care nursing purports to use simple, known technology, thereby avoiding the intrusiveness of modern technology. Both types of nursing deviate from nursing that is linked with the medical model: both focus on health rather than illness, on patients as active participants in care rather than recipients of care, and on sociocultural determinants as well as biologic determinants. Both primary nursing and primary health care nursing are the subject of international nursing research.

The importance of international research on nursing is exemplified by a comparative study of the processes of implementation and the perceptions of primary nursing in Australia, Japan, Belgium, the Netherlands, Norway, Canada, and the United States (Hegyvary, 1982). The major hypothesis explored was that primary nursing was related more to the degree and level of professionalization of nursing than to the cultural context in which nursing is practiced. Findings of the study were generalizable only to industrialized, modern countries whose per capita income and health services rank among the highest in the world. Although primary nursing is not a dominant method for organizing nursing or a definite trend in international nursing, where it is practiced the problems and the dilemmas of primary nursing are almost identical cross-nationally (Hegyvary, 1982). However, these problems were related more "to the characteristics of nursing practice than to the national system of health care or to social norms and values" (Hegyvary, 1982, pp. 174–175). Four future needs for the international advancement of professional nursing were identified by Hegyvary (1982): the need for defining practice, the need for research-based education of nurses, the need for nursing leadership, and the need for international cooperation, collegiality, and sharing. These findings well may represent similar needs in other countries.

One other study on primary health care nursing (Jaeger-Burns, 1981) qualifies as international nursing research as defined for this review. The investigator used six regional offices of WHO to facilitate the collaboration of the chief nurses of the Ministries of Health from 160 countries, which comprised the study sample; 34% of these responded during a 9-month period. The low response rate may call into question the study findings and interpretations. The findings may, however, provide nursing with rich qualitative data on perceptions and variations of the meaning and actual practice of community health nursing and primary health care nursing across nations. For primary health care nursing to respond to the needs of the population with particular consideration and attention to the economic and social values, there are the minimum requirements of promotion of safety, adequate nutrition, sanitation, maternal and child health care, control of endemic diseases, health education, proper treatment for common diseases, and the need for improving the educational preparation of nurses.

Alternatives to
Western Health Care Systems

In recent years many Western approaches to birth, such as hospital delivery, isolation of family members, anesthesiologic intervention during delivery, episiotomy, supination of patients, and lack of mobility during labor, have been questioned and other, older practices reconsidered. Some of the new and modern practices were formerly part of the Western health care system. This became apparent when beliefs and practices relating to childbirth in the United States were compared to those of other cultures. Cohen (1982) used a descriptive design and participant observation to describe beliefs and practices of childbirth in a black Carib village on the north coast of Honduras. Caribs are the native South American Indians living adjacent to the Caribbean Sea. Cohen's findings indicated that episiotomies were not done, expectant mothers were encouraged to walk throughout the delivery process, squatting was the preferred delivery method, delivery was a family affair, home delivery was the norm, and healers successfully helped one mother with postpartum psychosis. Although statistics on infant and maternal mortality were not readily available, perceptions of residents were of an almost total absence of maternal mortality. These findings support the alternative birthing practices that are being used increasingly in the United States.

Care of the institutionalized aged in the United States may also undergo some effective changes through consideration of similar care in other countries. A comparison of care of the institutionalized aged in Scotland and the United States revealed that the aged in Scotland were more pleased with their care than the aged in an American institution (Kayser-Jones, 1979). Criteria were more choice, freedom, independence, and institutional life more like life in the rest of society. Variables responsible for the disparity of such care were:

1. The financing and delivery of health care in (the U.S.) . . . which forces the elderly into dependency and stigmatizes them as "welfare patients," undeserving of high quality care.
2. A lack of leadership and responsibility by physicians and registered nurses for the care of the aged [in the United States]. (p. 198)

The Scottish had more appetizing food and varied activities, which they had some role in planning and they reported receiving more sensitive and experienced nursing care. In the above two studies researchers demonstrated that alternative models to the U.S. model of health care exist and that these models may be as effective as the U.S. model. Another researcher demonstrated the concurrent use of both trained and traditional healers (Gupta, 1978).

Nurses' Cultural Heritage
as an Independent Variable

Sociocultural variables influence individuals' expectations and responses to life events. Nurses as individuals are influenced by professional and societal values. Perceptions of the female nursing staffs of
two teaching hospitals ($n = 30$ in each; one U.S., one Indian) (Bhanumathi, 1977) found major differences related to level and degree of
self-care expected of patients and level of passivity/activity of patients
in hospitals. In the United States, with individualism, autonomy, and
independence as the prevailing societal normative values, nurses perceived patients as wanting to do all they could to get well and to
perform as many activities related to their care as possible. Indian
nurses, however, perceived their patients to be dependent and granted
them the expectation to be taken care of by others. "Others" invariably meant a doting and attentive circle of family members and friends,
and, therefore, the burden of care did not fall on the shoulders of the
nurses alone. The author speculated that the exemptions from normal
social role responsibilities articulated by Parsons (1951) are somewhat
incongruent with the expectations of U.S. nurses, but more congruent
with the expectations of Indian nurses. Also, Indian nurses perceived
mode of living and health habits as predominant causes of illness
(Bhanumathi, 1977).

Inferences about degree of suffering due to physical pain and
psychological distress have been investigated in six different nations
by Davitz, Davitz, and Higuchi (1977a, 1977b) and Davitz, Sameshima, and Davitz (1976). These investigators developed and used the
Standard Measure of the Inference of Suffering instrument, composed of 60 brief vignettes that describe illness or injury, its severity,
and the sex and age of patients. The findings were consistent among
cultures in rank order of illness categories, with highest significance
given to trauma, followed by infections, cardiovascular diseases, and
cancer; psychiatric illness was given the lowest ranking. This similarity
may reflect consistency in professional training. The two differences
that were reported supported the authors' hypothesis of anticipated
and inferred degree of suffering. Not surprisingly, the mean ratings
for psychological suffering of all six national groups were higher than
those perceived for physical pain. Two hypotheses that were supported
concerned nurses differing in their inferences of degree of suffering

from physical or psychological distress, and that there was an interaction of the concept of severity of a patient's illness with the cultural background of the nurse. Another significant finding was related to the variability in inferences among seemingly similar cultural groups: Koreans, Japanese, and Taiwanese. Similar variability may have been found among American subjects if cultural heritage had been considered as a research variable.

Major implications of these studies are that overt expression of pain may not be related necessarily to the severity of pain or to the psychological distress endured. Therefore, both objective and subjective measures of the degree and severity of pain are essential in assessment and diagnosis. These may be obtained through identification of normative pain expression within culture, through studies of expectations of severity of pain associated with different illnesses, and through intrusive procedures. The researchers also identified variables that influence nurses' judgments of severity of illnesses and injury, such as social class, patients' ethnic background, and the nurses' cultural background.

International Nursing Students

Studies about international students range from factors involved in recruiting them (Olesen & Davis, 1971) to responses of international students to the U.S. educational system (Abu-Saad, Kayser-Jones, & Gutierrez, 1982; Abu-Saad, Kayser-Jones, & Tien, 1982; Barnes, 1980; Kayser-Jones & Abu-Saad, 1982; Meleis, 1982a). The results of a survey (Abu-Saad & Kayser-Jones, 1981) of 82 foreign students in the United States indicated that stress during their educational experience stemmed mostly from faculty who were unfamiliar with foreign cultures and differences in values and social customs which contributed to the loneliness of the students.

Davitz, Davitz, and Sameshima (1976) qualitatively investigated the reactions and interactions of foreign and American nurses through the use of an open-ended interview. There were qualitative differences in role expectations, demonstrating the significance of culture in determining expectations, and potential misconceptions stemming from a lack of knowledge of different cultures. Those findings substantiated the significance of investigations using country of origin and cultural heritage as independent variables.

The Health of Women and the Family

One focus in international nursing studies has been women's health, specifically mothering, pregnancy, and family planning. This focus is understandable in light of foreign aid priorities to developing countries. International organizations such as WHO and U.S. Aid for International Development (USAID) identified maternal–child health and family planning as top priorities.

Of international concern is the unwarranted shift to bottle feeding, which has received minimal attention from nurse researchers. Many international nurses identified Western propaganda, indigenous beliefs, women working outside the home, lack of support to mothers, Western practices of rooming out, having bad or insufficient milk, and poor health of mothers as responsible for the preference of bottle feeding over breast-feeding (Drejer, 1980; India Nutrition Information Service, 1984; World Health Organization, 1979). Fear of cessation of milk may be another factor for the preference of bottle feeding. Ragheb and Smith (1979) identified beliefs and superstitions related to breast-feeding, as well as indigenous practices used by mothers to avoid cessation of breast milk. Though their sample was small and their design unclear, the findings provided nurses with acceptable strategies to enhance the flow of breast milk. On the other hand, others have found that mothers do not use the bottle for fear of cessation of breast milk (Houston, 1981).

International nursing research has helped to identify culturally bound syndromes as well as culturally specific responses to health and illness. For example, Israeli women identified with only 15 out of 47 symptoms perceived by Western women to be signs of premenstrual distress (Most, Woods, Dery, & Most, 1981). The authors speculated that the tremendous stress experienced by Israeli women due to political unrest may have overshadowed their perceptions of the premenstrual syndrome. However, because the authors also found that since there are varied meanings to the concept of stress in Hebrew, Western terminology for the signs of premenstrual distress may be equally suspect in explaining its lack of identification by Israeli women. If perceptions and meanings of stress and distress had been considered and identified in the context of the different cultures, the results may have been different.

That responses and meanings differ is demonstrated in a study to identify attachment and bonding behaviors of mothers in Egypt (Govaerts & Patino, 1981). Though this study also included Western-generated constructs, the findings indicated that some behaviors transcended cultures, such as smiling and enfacing, and other behaviors were culture-specific and molded by the environment, such as kissing, patting, and encompassing. While using a familiar Western attachment framework provided the impetus for the development of the behavioral checklist, the use of descriptive and qualitative designs allowed the discovery of the centrality of the extended family in labor and delivery and the early incorporation of the newborn into the family system. In some cultures, the infant is expected to be molded to fit into the family unit (Caudill & Weinstein, 1969; Govaerts & Patino, 1981) rather than as is a prevailing expectation in the United States, the family accepting the individuality and uniqueness of the infant. This is demonstrated in studies that support sensitive mothering and the need for responsiveness of mothers to infant cues (Ainsworth, 1979; Kayiatos, Adams, & Gilman, 1984).

That the family is central in the care of people also was documented in a collaborative international study based on investigations completed in the United States. In comparing an Egyptian and an American sample of oncology patients, Lindsey, Ahmed, and Dodd (1985) demonstrated that the Egyptian sample had "more contact and longer duration of relationship with their identified network" (p. 41), listed more network members, had a higher mean total functional component, and had the largest proportion of their social support network as family and relatives. Therefore, families expect to participate in the care of patients (Leke, 1982) and could be incorporated easily into the care of their hospitalized relatives (Eldar & Eldar, 1984).

Development of
Assessment and Research Tools

One value inherent in international research lies in the kind of questions the findings may help to answer on the national scene. International samples provide a potentially broadened, greater range of behaviors than samples of studies conducted in a single sociocultural context. For example, Brink (1984) used Kluckhohn's value orientation schedules (1950, 1951, 1953) to develop a value assessment tool and tested it on the Annang of Nigeria. The testing of the tool in a single rather homogeneous culture allowed the development of a data analysis technique that can be used by all who may wish to assess value orientation. Brink's research, besides increasing an understanding of value orientation of the Annang of Nigeria, also validated the potential use of the assessment tool for the many subcultures within the United States.

International studies can also uncover biases inherent in some Western diagnostic tools designed for middle-class white Americans and in turn may lead to the development of culturally sensitive tools. Two studies of international samples demonstrated the cultural bias of a diagnostic tool used frequently in nursing. In a pilot study, Olade (1984) tested the Denver Developmental Screening Test (DDST) on a convenience sample of 94 children ranging in age from 1 month to 6 years who came with their mothers to prenatal clinics in Ibadan, Nigeria. Her study lent validity to the significance of the test in the early detection of children at risk for developmental handicaps in developing countries; thus, her findings could benefit other nations. However, the study confirmed the lack of sensitivity of the test to the sociocultural and economic backgrounds or the lifestyles of the children. This finding should lead American nurses to more cautious use of the tool because color tests, games, and toys can only be standardized within socioculturally and economically compatible groups.

Sample size was not a significant issue in another international study of 6000 subjects, which was aimed at establishing normative values with which to compare clients from other countries to the United States. Williams (1984) reported on the use of the DDST with children in Metro-Manila (Philippines) to determine the characteristics of low and high scoring children. The results indicated that the Metro-Manila sample attained a majority of the items much later than the American samples. Most of the items were ambiguous or inappropriate for children in the Philippines, based on Williams' delineation of items not passed by 90% of the sample. Discriminant analysis showed that the care of mothers or of mother-substitutes was associated significantly with children's performances. Another cluster was related to the mother, her level of education, and her birthplace. Implications of the study pointed to the significance of the home environment and of the caregivers of children in the extended family in the Philippines (Williams, 1984).

TRENDS IN INTERNATIONAL
NURSING RESEARCH

It is apparent from the studies reviewed for this chapter that while international nursing research is in a beginning phase, definite trends are emerging. Investigation themes were:

1. Professional concerns: Image, status, role of nursing and nurses, immigration of nurses, and roles of indigenous workers in health care of nations;
2. Educational concerns: Types of educational programs most effective in preparing nurses from other nations, recruitment, and retention of students and graduates;
3. Women's health: Determinants and responses of women to such universal events as birthing, mothering, menstruating, and lactating;
4. Family concerns: Roles of family in support, care, and development of its members;
5. Culture and country of origin: As independent variables in responses of nurses and patients to health and illness events;
6. Clinical therapeutics as practiced in other nations or cultures: Range, types, and levels of effectiveness.

The trends demonstrate a shift from nurse-focused research to patient-focused research. Although there are a number of ethnographic studies and some phenomenologic studies related to universal professional and educational concerns, there are no reviews that synthesize these concerns regionally or worldwide, or outline future studies. The International Council of Nurses could be a medium for synthesis and development of future studies.

There still exists a severe gap in knowledge of indigenous health care practices. The use of alternative clinical therapeutics could more readily be studied in other countries because these therapeutics might be more congruent with these cultures. For example, Locsin (1981) studied the effect of music on the pain experience of postoperative patients in the Philippines. Prakasamma and Bhaduri (1984) demonstrated that the use of one form of Indian yoga (Pranayam) helped to expand the lungs of patients with pleural effusion after aspiration of liquids. Once the properties of the culture-specific nursing therapeutics and their effectiveness are established, they can be exported for testing cross-nationally, or vice versa.

Few studies published in U.S. journals by nurse researchers from other countries have samples from those countries; examples include studies by Adler (1969), Bergman (1964), and Cordiner and Hall (1971). A limited view of what constitutes research, based on criteria derived from a traditional view of science that has dominated nursing, may have decreased the probability of publication of foreign research in U.S. journals. Equally scarce are publications by nurses or other researchers from the United States who conducted research abroad and published the results in nursing journals. Few researchers have been able to do so (Kayser-Jones, 1979; Olade, 1984; Williams, 1984).

FUTURE RESEARCH

Although the significance of international research has been discussed (de Chesnay, 1983; Meleis, 1985), there have been almost no published articles reviewing and critiquing methodology in international nursing research. Considering that many of the studies used multilingual instruments, modified tools to fit different cultures, and various means of collecting data for similar designs cross-nationally, the authors most probably had to resort to innovative approaches to data collection. Extensive accounts of these issues, as well as strategies for culture-specific data collection methods, would be useful additions for nursing literature. It would be helpful also to know how authors establish equivalency of the translated instruments and tools.

The choice of research questions for an investigation, the meaning of the constructs under investigation, and the selection of culturally appropriate instruments, as well as data interpretation, are subject to etic and emic meanings. Future investigations as well as clinical practice can benefit from published dialogues regarding the varied meanings. An example is the meaning of premenstrual distress by Israeli women; their health care providers may help to shed some light on its perceived absence by these women (Most, Woods, Dery, & Most, 1981). The finding that Egyptian cancer patients do not include health care professionals in their support systems is a curious finding in light of findings in the United States that patients invariably list and consider health care professionals as being within their social support repertoire (Lindsey, Ahmed, & Dodd, 1985; Williams, 1984). The elucidation of these findings through other investigations will be necessary for developing knowledge related to central propositions in nursing.

Several studies reported here utilized existing international structures and organizations to facilitate data collection. These organizations have demonstrated willingness to assist in such research endeavors, but their resources have been far better utilized by other professionals. A data base of investigative areas in nursing may be helpful in attracting nurse researchers to collaborate in exploring research areas of universal interest. ICN, WHO, and some U.S. organizations may be able to help develop and publish strategies on how to utilize these international organizations to enhance international nursing research. International organizational commitment to nursing research needs to be reaffirmed periodically (Glass, 1977) as a reminder to nurses to engage in international collaborative research.

In cross-national research, one of the most pressing issues is the comparability of the sample. Variables most often used in the United States to establish comparability are occupation, education, and income. These may not be useful in all cultures; other variables would be lineage, tribe, or occupational prestige. Similarly, the concept of urbanization for one country has a different meaning for another, and therefore level of urbanization may be more appropriate than urbanization as a nominal variable. International nursing researchers of the future should consider these variations and address how these variations should be controlled.

Convenience samples and low survey response rates represent the state of the art in international research. Strategies are needed that begin with acceptance of this situation and that creatively develop means of decreasing error and increasing generalizability; for example, defining the sample characteristics carefully and comparing them to other available data may achieve an increase in generalizability. Theoretical sampling may be more appropriate at times, whereas requesting the view of local scientists on how representative a sample is may be appropriate at other times. Careful selection of the convenience sample and paying attention to variables identified in other research may also enhance generalizability. There is a need for methodological papers that begin with the state of the art and proceed to develop useful strategies. Pilot studies also may help identify the most significant variables in culturally specific sampling.

Low survey return prompted some researchers (Styles, 1984) to rely on other primary and secondary sources of data. The use of several samples and sources is likely to provide more reliable data and more contextually imbedded research. In trying to answer questions related to whether international nursing is a speciality, and to its major concepts and research questions, Henkle (1979) used a multiplicity of data sources and methodologies. She reviewed literature, interviewed nurse administrators of international agencies, and sent questionnaires to preselected nurses with extensive international backgrounds and to a random sample of 78 American nurses working abroad who were sponsored by international organizations. She identified nine areas that constitute the domain of international nursing and concluded that the results indicate conflicting views on whether international nursing is a specialization or not. The sampling process and the variables on which the sample was selected were appropriate for the purpose of the study.

The ethics of international nursing research and the resulting ethical dilemmas, including varied meanings or definitions of volunteerism, coercion, and consent process, have received minimal attention (Meleis, 1980a). Identifying issues and varied strategies in collecting data while preserving the rights of the individual as well as of the country could enhance international research.

STRATEGIES FOR
CUMULATIVE INVESTIGATIONS

Reviews designed to address the state of the art in any of the above six areas of concern also are needed. Reviews focused on specific regions or countries could help to identify areas of future investigation. For example, a review of the published writings based on survey, phenomenological, and descriptive designs of one region such as the Middle East (Meleis, 1979a, 1979b, 1979c, 1979d, 1980b, 1982b; Meleis & Burton, 1981; Meleis, El-Sanabary, & Beeson, 1979; Meleis & Hassan, 1980; Pattison, 1984; Siassi & Fozouni, 1982) may be useful for understanding the cultural context and identifying potential future research areas. Similar reviews for other regions also would be useful.

Other strategies would be those designed to enhance collaborative research. Studies could be initiated in the United States and replicated abroad, providing a potential for comparison. For example, Davitz (1972) used the critical incident technique to identify stressful situations as perceived by students in a Nigerian school of nursing. Her study replicated one undertaken in the United States (Fox & Diamond, 1965) and, therefore, provided an opportunity for comparative methodological analysis. Such collaborative efforts are feasible particularly because nurses are the largest group of U.S. health care professionals engaged in international health practices and activities (Baker, Weisman, & Piwoz, 1984).

Certain ongoing national research could benefit from comparisons with internationally conceived and implemented research studies. If data banks are developed to house ongoing U.S. research studies, international colleagues may elect to join and collaborate in such studies. Either existing organizations or new international research institutes developed for this purpose could act as data banks and facilitate international research.

International organizations may identify certain research needs and ask key persons to collaborate in an international investigation. Other professionals have used this strategy, and more recently it has been used by nursing divisions in international organizations. A case in point is a project on the regulation of nursing that was initiated in 1983 to help the ICN organization develop a position on the future in regulation of nursing education and practice. The results of this extensive worldwide study, which relied on examination and analysis of primary and secondary data sources, are presented in the form of 12 principles. These principles, in the words of the author, "represent a proposal for a fundamental code regarding regulation of the professions" (Styles, 1984, p. 102). These principles emerged from a study of existing regulations and were disseminated to the world of nursing at the International Council of Nursing meeting in Israel in 1985.

A group of researchers with an area of investigation of universal interest may plan a subject-specific international conference to share findings and to promote the development of other collaborative international investigations. For the success of such a conference in promulgating a collaborative approach, more than one institution should participate, preferably an international institution. To simplify the mechanics of cosponsoring an international research conference, one such conference was attached to the ICN conference in 1985. The planners, Norbeck, Minaim, and Krulik, representing universities in the United States, Japan, and Israel, secured sponsorship from the universities. A request for identification of persons interested in social support research was followed by a request for research papers. The results of this correspondence yielded a useful model to be followed by others who are interested in international research. Besides the pre-ICN research conference on social support, which included two days of exchange of research findings on social support from different parts of the world, a directory was generated with names of those who are internationally interested in social support, and a bibiography was compiled of studies published by nurses on social support and social networks (J. Norbeck, personal communication, April, 1985). This is a very useful model for the promotion of international nursing research.

Results of international nursing research can provide nations with some valid guidelines for their nursing profession and nurse practice. International nursing research also can provide us with the sensitivity needed to supply care to the multiplicity of ethnic groups in our midst. Most important, international nursing research could provide an arena for testing competing hypotheses under diverse but natural cultural conditions, the means to develop a whole gamut of perceptions and responses to health and illness, and insight into the varied meanings of constructs and experiences related to nursing care. Nursing knowledge in some areas could develop by leaps and bounds if the pursuit of its investigations were organized internationally.

REFERENCES

Abu-Saad, H., & Kayser-Jones, J. (1981). Foreign nursing students in the U.S.A.: Problems in their educational experiences. *Journal of Advanced Nursing, 6,* 397–403.
Abu-Saad, H., Kayser-Jones, J., & Gutierrez, Y. (1982). Latin American nursing

students in the United States. *Journal of Nursing Education, 21*(7), 16–21.

Abu-Saad, H., Kayser-Jones, J., & Tien, J. (1982). Asian nursing students in the United States. *Journal of Nursing Education, 21*(7), 11–15.

Adler, S. P. (1969). Swedish student nurses: A descriptive study. *Nursing Research, 18*, 363–365.

Ainsworth, M. D. S. (1979). Infant–mother attachment. *American Psychologist, 34*, 932–937.

Bachu, A. (1973). Indian nurses in the United States. *International Nursing Review, 20*, 114–116, 122.

Baker, T. D., Weisman, D., & Piwoz, E. (1984). United States health professionals in international health work. *American Journal of Public Health, 74*, 438–441.

Barnes, S. Y. (1980). Problems foreign nurses encounter in passing psychiatric nursing on U.S. exams for licensure. *Journal of Nursing Education, 19*(1), 19–25.

Baudrey, J. (1978). The nurse and the medical assistant: Functions and status. *International Nursing Review, 25*, 108–112.

Beck, F. S. (1965). The family's part in caring for the patient. *International Nursing Review, 12*(1), 31–50.

Bergman, R. L. (1964). Team nursing in public health in Israel. *Nursing Research, 13*, 72–74.

Bergman, R. L., Krulik, T., & Ditzian, I. (1976). Opinion on nursing. *International Nursing Review, 23*, 15–24.

Bhanumathi, P. P. (1977). Nurses' conceptions of "sick role" and "good patient" behaviour: A cross-cultural comparison. *International Nursing Review, 24*, 20–24.

Brink, P. J. (1984). Value orientation as an assessment tool in cultural diversity. *Nursing Research, 33*, 198–203.

Bryant, J. H. (1980). WHO's program of health for all by the year 2000: A macro system for health policy. A challenge to social science research. *Social Science and Medicine, 14A*, 381–386.

Caudill, W., & Weinstein, H. (1969). Maternal care and infant behavior in Japan and America. *Psychiatry, 32*, 12–43.

Cohen, F. S. (1982). Childbirth belief and practice in a Garifuna (Black Carib) village on the north coast of Honduras. *Western Journal of Nursing Research, 4*, 193–208.

Collière, M. F. (1980). Development of primary health care. *International Nursing Review, 27*, 169–172.

Cordiner, C. M., & Hall, D. J. (1971). The use of the motivational analysis test in the selection of Scottish nursing students. *Nursing Research, 20*, 356–362.

Croog, S. H., & Caudill, W., & Blumen, J. L. (1968). Value orientations, religious identity, and career decisions of nursing students in Japan. *Nursing Research, 17*, 161–166.

Davitz, L. L. (1976). Foreign and American nurses: Reactions and interactions. *Nursing Outlook, 24*, 237–242.

Davitz, L. L., & Davitz, J. R., & Higuchi, Y. (1977a). Cross-cultural inferences of physical pain and psychological distress—1. *Nursing Times, 73*, 521–523.

Davitz, L. L., Davitz, J. R., & Higuchi, Y. (1977b). Cross-cultural inferences of physical pain and psychological distress—2. *Nursing Times, 73*, 556–558.

Davitz, L. L., Davitz, J. R., & Sameshima, Y. (1972). Identification of stressful situations in a Nigerian school of nursing. *Nursing Research, 21*, 352–357.

Davitz, L. L., Sameshima, Y., & Davitz, J. R. (1976). Suffering as viewed in six different cultures. *American Journal of Nursing, 76*, 1296–1297.

deCastro, I. B., Lunardi, N., Coloriti, A. M., & de Moura, F. (1976). Changes in the image of the nurse in Brazil. *International Nursing Review, 23*, 43–47.

deChesnay, M. (1983). Cross-cultural research: Advantages and disadvantages. *International Nursing Review, 30*, 21–23.

Drejer, G. F. (1980). Bottle feeding in Douala, Cameroons. *Journal of Tropical Pediatrics, 26*(1), 31–36.

Eldar, R., & Eldar, E. (1984). A place for the family in hospital life. *International Nursing Review, 31*, 40–42.

Fox, D. J., & Diamond, L. K. (1964). *Satisfying and stressful situations in basic programs in nursing education.* New York: Teachers College, Columbia University.

Glass, H. P. (1977). Research: An international perspective. *Nursing Research, 26*, 230–236.

Govaerts, K., & Patino, E. (1981). Attachment behavior of the Egyptian mother. *International Journal of Nursing Studies, 18*, 53–60.

Gupta, K. (1978). Qualified personnel or traditional midwives? Women's choice in rural India. *International Nursing Review, 25*, 175–181.

Hegyvary, S. T. (1982). *The change to primary nursing: A cross-cultural view of professional nursing practice.* St. Louis: Mosby.

Henkle, J. O. (1979). International nursing: A specialty? *International Nursing Review, 26*, 170–173.

Hentinen, M. (1983). Need for instruction and support of the wives of patients with myocardial infarction. *Journal of Advanced Nursing, 8*, 519–524.

Houston, M. J. (1981). Breast feeding: Success or failure. *Journal of Advanced Nursing, 6*, 447–454.

India Nutrition Information Service. (1984). Breast feeding versus bottle feeding. *Nursing Journal of India, 75*(2), 32–33.

Jaeger-Burns, J. (1981). The relationship of nursing to primary health care internationally. *International Nursing Review, 28*, 167–175.

Jato, M., Mounlom, D., Colgate, S., & Carrière, J. (1979). Adapting nursing textbooks for Africa: A necessity. *International Nursing Review, 26*, 21–23.

Kayiatos, R., Adams, J., & Gilman, B. (1984). The arrival of a rival: Maternal perceptions of toddlers' regressive behaviors after the birth of a sibling. *Journal of Nurse-Midwifery, 29*(3), 205–213.

Kayser-Jones, J. (1979). Care of the institutionalized aged in Scotland and the United States: A comparative study. *Western Journal of Nursing Research, 1*, 191–199.

Kayser-Jones, J. S., & Abu-Saad, H. (1982). Loneliness: Its relationship to the educational experience of international nursing students in the United States. *Western Journal of Nursing Research, 4*, 301–315.

Kelly, M. A. (1973). Beliefs of Iranian nurses and nursing students about nurses and nursing education. *International Nursing Review, 20*, 108–111.

Kleczkowski, B. (1980). Matching goals and health care systems: An international perspective. *Social Science and Medicine, 14A*, 391–395.

Kluckhorn, F. R. (1950). Dominant and substitute profiles of cultural orientations. *Social Forces, 28*, 375–394.

Kluckhorn, F. R. (1951). Dominant and variant cultural value orientations. *Social*

Welfare Forum, 77, 97–113.

Kluckhorn, F. R. (1953). Dominant and variant value orientations. In C. Kluckhorn & H. A. Murray (Eds.), *Personality in nature, society and culture* (2nd ed.) (pp. 342–357). New York: Knopf.

Kruse, M., & Munck, H. (1965). Conditions of work of nurses in the northern European countries. *International Nursing Review, 12*(2), 50–55.

Leke, J. T. (1982). The problem of availability of drugs in hospitals: The example of Makurdi, Nigeria. *International Nursing Review, 29*, 46–47.

Lindsey, A. M., Ahmed, N., & Dodd, M. J. (1985) Social support: Network and quality as perceived by Egyptian cancer patients. *Cancer Nursing, 8*, 37–42.

Locsin, R. (1981). The effect of music on the pain of selected post-operative patients. *Journal of Advanced Nursing, 6*, 19–25.

Logan, W. (1980). The migration of nursing personnel. *International Nursing Review, 27*(4), 119–122.

Mejia, A., Pizurki, H., & Royston, E. (1979). *Physician and nurse migration: Analysis and policy implications: A report of a WHO study*. Geneva: World Health Organization.

Meleis, A. I. (1979a). The development of a conceptually based nursing curriculum: An international experiment. *Journal of Advanced Nursing, 4*, 659–671.

Meleis, A. I. (1979b). The graduate dilemma: The Kuwaiti experience. *International Journal of Nursing Studies, 16*, 337–343.

Meleis, A. I. (1979c). The health care system of Kuwait: The social paradoxes. *Social Science and Medicine, 13A*, 743–749.

Meleis, A. I. (1979d). International issues in nursing education: The case of Kuwait. *International Nursing Review, 26*, 107–110.

Meleis, A. I. (1980a). Cross-cultural research. In A. J. Davis & J. C. Krueger (Eds.), *Patients, nurses, ethics* (pp. 137–147). New York: American Journal of Nursing Company.

Meleis, A. I. (1980b). A model for establishment of educational programmes in developing countries: The nursing paradoxes in Kuwait. *Journal of Advanced Nursing, 5*, 285–300.

Meleis, A. I. (1982a). Arab students in western universities: Social properties and dilemmas. *Journal of Higher Education, 53*(4), 439–447.

Meleis, A. I. (1982b). Effect of modernization on Kuwaiti women. *Social Science and Medicine, 16*, 965–970.

Meleis, A. I. (1985). International research for knowledge development. *Nursing Outlook, 33*, 144–147.

Meleis, A. I., & Burton, P. S. (1981). Innovative educational changes: A paradigm. *International Journal of Nursing Studies, 18*, 33–39.

Meleis, A. I., El-Sanabary, N., & Beeson, D. (1979). Women, modernization, and education in Kuwait. *Comparative Education Review, 23*(1), 115–124.

Meleis, A. I., & Hassan, S. H. (1980). Oil rich, nurse poor: The nursing crisis in the Persian Gulf. *Nursing Outlook, 28*, 238–243.

Most, A. F., Woods, N. F., Dery, G. K., & Most, B. M. (1981). Distress associated with menstruation among Israeli women. *International Journal of Nursing Studies, 18*, 61–71.

Olade, R. A. (1984). Evaluation of the Denver developmental screening test as applied to African children. *Nursing Research, 33*, 204–207.

Olesen, V., & Davis, A. J. (1971). Preliminary findings on factors in the recruitment of foreign students. *Nursing Research, 20,* 159–162.

Parsons, T. (1951). *The social system.* London: The Free Press of Glencoe.

Pattison, E. M. (1984). War and mental health in Lebanon. *Journal of Operational Psychiatry, 15,* 13–38.

Prakasamma, M., & Bhaduri, A. (1984). A study of yoga as a nursing intervention in the care of patients with pleural effusion. *Journal of Advanced Nursing, 9,* 127–133.

Ragheb, S., & Smith, E. W. (1979). Beliefs and customs regarding breast feeding among Egyptian women in Alexandria. *International Journal of Nursing Studies, 16,* 73–83.

Ronaghy, H. A., Zeighami, B., Agah, T., Rouhani, R., & Zimmer, S. P. (1975). Migration of Iranian nurses to the U.S.: A study of one school of nursing in Iran. *International Nursing Review, 22,* 87–88.

Siassi, I., & Fozouni, B. (1982). Psychiatry and the elderly in the Middle East: A report from Iran. *International Journal of Aging and Human Development, 15*(2), 107–120.

Styles, M. (1984). *Project on the regulation of nursing, 1984.* Geneva: International Council of Nurses.

Williams, P. D. (1984). The Metro-Manila developmental screening test: A normative study. *Nursing Research, 33,* 208–212.

World Health Organization. (1979). *Collaborative Study on breast-feeding.* Geneva: Author.

World Health Organization/United Nations International Children's Fund. (1978). *Alma Ata: Primary health care.* Geneva: World Health Organization.

Chapter 10

Conceptual Models
of Nursing

MARY CIPRIANO SILVA
SCHOOL OF NURSING
GEORGE MASON UNIVERSITY

CONTENTS

The purpose of this review was to summarize and assess research related to five conceptual models of nursing, with particular emphasis on identifying how the models were used in the research. The following conceptual models of nursing were included: the Johnson Behavioral System Model (1968, 1980), the Roy Adaptation Model (1970, 1976, 1984), the Orem Self-Care Model (1971, 1980, 1985), the Ro-

Preparation of this chapter was funded by Rita Carty, Dean, School of Nursing, George Mason University, and by the Epsilon Zeta Chapter of Sigma Theta Tau, George Mason University, Fairfax, Virginia.

    The author thanks the editors, Joyce J. Fitzpatrick, and Roma Lee Taunton, and Advisory Board member Susan R. Gortner for their helpful comments on a draft of this chapter. She also acknowledges the help of Jeanne Sorrell with hand searches of the literature and Patricia Hawley with technical preparation of the manuscript. Finally, she expresses deep appreciation to the five nurse theorists mentioned herein who, through the professional sharing of their nursing models, made this chapter possible.

gers Science of Unitary Human Beings Model (1970, 1980, 1983), and the Newman Health Model (1979). These models were included because investigators have generated more current empirical research from them than other nursing models. The review begins with a summary of retrieval strategies and criteria used for inclusion of the studies and the models. Next, studies in which each of the five models were used are summarized and assessed. Finally, strengths, weaknesses, and future directions regarding the use of nursing models in research are identified.

To locate research related to conceptual models of nursing, systematic hand searches of the literature were done on every article in *Nursing Research* (1952 – 1984), *International Journal of Nursing Studies* (1963 – 1984), *Research in Nursing and Health* (1978 – 1984), *Advances in Nursing Science* (1978 – 1984), and *Western Journal of Nursing Research* (1979 – 1984). Hand searches of the literature also were done on 39 known nursing theory books and other relevant research documents, such as the proceedings of the American Nurses' Association's nine research conferences (1967 – 1974). In addition, four MEDLINE searches (1971 – 1984) using four different key words and a computerized *Cumulative Index to Nursing and Allied Health Literature* search (1983 – 1984) were conducted. Finally, each of the five nurse theorists included herein was asked to review a draft of the chapter for accuracy and completeness.

To delimit this review, the following criteria for inclusion of the studies were specified: (a) The study must be published, empirical research, explicitly related to a conceptual model of nursing, and (b) the study must be of sufficient breadth and depth to be critiqued. Nonempirical research (e.g., reviews of the literature and research critiques and commentaries) was eliminated because of the emphasis within the chapter on data-generating studies. Abstracts were eliminated because of their insufficient breadth and depth for critiquing, and unpublished works such as paper presentations, masters' theses, and doctoral dissertations were eliminated because of space requirements, retrieval difficulties, and lack of formal peer review.

Criteria for inclusion of the conceptual models of nursing also were specified as follows: (a) The model must have generated at least six published empirical studies of sufficient breadth and depth, and (b) the majority of the studies must have been published between 1974 and 1984. Limitations of the review included the difficulty in locating studies related to conceptual models of nursing and the difficulty in defining and operationalizing the criteria for the inclusion of the studies and the models.

RESEARCH BASED ON THE
JOHNSON BEHAVIORAL SYSTEM MODEL

In Dorothy E. Johnson's Behavioral System Model (1980), persons are viewed as behavioral systems composed of seven subsystems: attachment, dependency, ingestive, eliminative, sexual, aggressive, and achievement. When these behavioral systems are functioning effectively in meeting subsystem goals, the systems are in balance; when these behavioral systems are functioning ineffectively in meeting subsystem goals, these systems are in imbalance. The nurse's role is to foster effective and efficient behavioral functioning.

Investigators have reported the use of the Johnson model as a basis for research since 1974. Using this model, Holaday (1974) studied whether chronically ill children showed different achievement behaviors than well children and found different response trends between the two groups. In 1981 and 1982, Holaday again used the Johnson model, albeit briefly, as one of several theoretical frameworks for studying 388 chronically ill infants' crying bouts and 6 mothers' responses to this crying. These data were compared to data on crying bouts and maternal responses to this crying in a literature control group of 26 well infants and their mothers. Several differences were found between the crying patterns of ill and well infants, although maternal responses to the crying of ill and well children were similar. In these three studies, Holaday could have strengthened the use of the Johnson model in her research by more explicit integration of the model throughout her studies.

Investigators also have used the Johnson model to study visually impaired children (Small, 1980), patients with posttransfusion hepatitis (Damus, 1980), and children with leukemia (Lovejoy, 1983). Although the model was not integrated into the research in the Small study, the author emphasized that it could guide practice for visually impaired children. Damus stressed that a tool derived from the model worked well in assessing patients with posttransfusion hepatitis; however, she reported no information on the tool's construction or on its reliability or validity. Lovejoy, in studying leukemic children's perceptions of family behaviors, found that they perceived problems in four of the subsystems associated with the Johnson model. However, like Damus, Lovejoy reported no validity or reliability data on her instrument, but she acknowledged that these data were needed.

Several investigators (Bruce et al., 1980; Derdiarian, 1983; Derdiarian & Forsythe, 1983; Majesky, Brester, & Nishio, 1978) used the Johnson model primarily as the basis for tool construction. After a thorough review of the literature and multiple pilot tests, Majesky et al. (1978) developed a tool to measure quality of nursing care. These investigators established content validity of the tool, performed an item analysis, and computed split-half and interrater reliabilities. Although the tool was constructed with care, the relationship between it and the Johnson model was not described clearly.

Bruce et al. (1980) developed a tool to measure outcome criteria for fluid and electrolyte balance in persons with end-stage renal disease. They used the achievement, ingestive, and eliminative subsystems of the Johnson model, with the latter two subsystems combined, as the organizing framework for the tool. Although the investigators reported content validity, it was unclear how reliability data were obtained or how the 94 criteria of the tool were classified into the subsystems of the Johnson model.

Derdiarian (1983) and Derdiarian and Forsythe (1983) furthered the work of Majesky et al. (1978) and Bruce et al. (1980) by implementing a systematic and comprehensive process for development of a tool based on the Johnson model. The tool, which measured perceived behavioral changes of adult cancer patients, was organized around the subsystems associated with the model. The authors' careful attention to measurement helped to ensure the tool's validity and reliability. Despite this strength, Derdiarian intentionally chose not to discuss the relationship of the tool to the propositions of the model.

RESEARCH BASED ON THE
ROY ADAPTATION MODEL

In Sister Callista Roy's Adaptation Model (1984), persons are viewed as adaptive systems with regulator and cognator control processes that manifest themselves through four effector modes: physiologic, self-concept, role function, and interdependence. The nurse's role is to modify the outcome of these adaptive systems by increasing persons' adaptive responses and decreasing their ineffective responses.

Investigators have reported use of the Roy model as a basis for research since 1975. Leonard (1975) alluded to the Roy model in discussing the nursing care implications of psychiatric patients' attitudes toward nursing interventions. She conjectured that the model could assist in desirable manipulation of environmental stimuli.

In 1977, Nolan used the Roy model, along with other theoretical frameworks, to study nursing interventions in the operating room. Her hypothesis that 50 sedated presurgical patients who received a systematic nursing intervention would recall more positive items postoperatively than 50 sedated presurgical patients who received routine nursing care was supported. Although this study had several methodological limitations such as lack of random assignment, the author appropriately used the model as a basis for the nursing intervention. In another study occurring in an acute care setting, Guzzetta (1979) alluded to the Roy model as one of her theoretical frameworks in determining the relationship between learning and stress in postcoronary care unit patients. In this methodologically sound study, the theoretical framework of adaptation could have been identified more systematically throughout the study.

A few investigators (Fawcett, 1981a, 1981b; Kehoe, 1981) used the Roy model to focus on the cesarean experience. Using an open-ended questionnaire, Fawcett (1981a) studied the reaction of 24 parents to cesarean birth. She classified responses within the four modes of the Roy model by using content analysis and found that both mothers and fathers expressed need deficits in all modes. Fawcett integrated the Roy model well throughout her study but did not describe how she classified responses within each of the four modes to ensure their independence. In a derivative publication, Fawcett (1981b) elaborated on the reactions of cesarean fathers.

The Kehoe (1981) research was focused on identifying the nursing needs of 11 postpartum mothers who had experienced unexpected cesarean births. Like Fawcett (1981a, 1981b), Kehoe used content analysis to organize the data around the four modes of the Roy model. Based on the data, she concluded that postpartum cesarean mothers have unique nursing needs. A limitation of the study was the difficulty Kehoe had in classifying the postpartum mothers' responses into each of the four modes so that the response did not overlap.

Another study that was focused on classifying data into the

modes of the Roy model was conducted by C. E. Smith, Garvis, and Martinson (1983). To elicit needs of parents whose children were newly diagnosed with cancer, C. E. Smith et al. used content analysis to analyze interview data. Unlike the preceding study, trained nurse raters found it possible to sort parent messages into one of the four modes of the Roy model, with agreement ranging from 82% to 100%. This high interrater reliability is encouraging for other investigators choosing to organize their data around the modes of the Roy Adaptation Model.

Other investigators (Farkas, 1981; Norris, Campbell, & Brenkert, 1982) also used one or more modes of the Roy model to organize their research. Farkas compared adaptation problems of elderly persons who were on waiting lists for admission to nursing homes to those of elderly persons who had not applied for such admission. She found few signficant differences between the two groups, although adaptation problems in the physiologic mode appeared to be the catalyst that initiated the nursing home application. Using a transcutaneous oxygen monitor, Norris et al. focused only on the physiologic mode and studied the effect of three focal stimuli, suctioning, repositioning, or performing a heelstick, on the blood oxygen levels in 25 premature infants. They found that transcutaneous oxygen did not decrease significantly during the heelstick but did so during repositioning and suctioning, with suctioning placing the infants at the highest risk for maladaptive responses due to hypoxemia. The investigators conducted a methodologically sound study and integrated the Roy model throughout.

In an example of theory testing generated from clinical observations, Hammond, Roberts, and Silva (1983) questioned the implicit assumption within the Roy model that both first- and second-level assessment data are necessary to make accurate nursing diagnoses. First-level assessment data refer to information gathered about behaviors in each of the Roy modes; second-level assessment data refer to identification of focal, contextual, and residual factors that influence the behaviors of concern. The investigators hypothesized as follows: Among 29 nurses familiar with the Roy model, those nurses using first-level assessment data would make as many accurate nursing diagnoses as those nurses using both first- and second-level assessment data. The hypothesis was supported, suggesting that an assumption of the Roy model may be invalid. However, this conclusion must be tempered by the small sample size and the difficulty in operationally defining accurate nursing diagnoses.

In addition to the preceding studies, the Roy model also was used as a framework for tool development (Ide, 1978; Lewis, Firsich, & Parsell, 1979). Based on the modes of the Roy model, Ide developed a tool to measure self-perceived adaptation level regarding one's internal and external environment in noninstitutionalized persons 65 years of age and older. The steps Ide took to ensure validity and reliability were unclear, although she noted that the scale could be used both in nursing research and practice. Lewis et al. also developed a tool based on the modes of the Roy model. The tool, designed to measure health outcomes of nursing care for adult patients on chemotherapy, was composed of a form that was focused on patient background variables and a questionnaire that was composed of five scales measuring patients' self-reported physical and emotional well-being. The investigators assessed both validity and reliability of the measures and, based on the results, recommended clinical use of some of the scales and refinement of others. Although attention was paid to validity and reliability, the use of the Roy model as an organizing framework throughout all phases of tool development was unclear.

RESEARCH BASED ON THE OREM SELF-CARE MODEL

In Dorothea E. Orem's Self-Care Model (1985), persons are viewed as possessing self-care agency. Self-care agency is one's ability for engaging in self-care. When self-care agency is not adequate to meet therapeutic self-care demands, self-care deficits occur. The nurse's role is to design nursing systems that assist persons with self-care deficits to maximize self-care and improve health.

As early as 1971, Allison briefly noted the Orem model as a theoretical framework in a study on the meaning of rest. More recently, the Orem model was cited briefly in a variety of research (Chang, Uman, Linn, Ware, & Kane, 1984; Dickson & Lee-Villasenor, 1982; Dodd, 1982, 1983, 1984; Karl, 1982; Leatt, Bay, & Stinson, 1981; Rothlis, 1984; Tompkins, 1980; Toth, 1980). The Orem's model was developed in more depth in clinical nursing research focused on patients with diabetes (Miller, 1982), hypertension (Harper, 1984), and cancer (Kubricht, 1984).

Using an investigator-designed self-care tool, Miller (1982) evaluated the self-care agency of 65 ambulatory adult patients with diabetes. She recorded these data on a care plan based on the Orem concepts of self-care deficits and self-care requisites. Using grounded theory methodology, she eventually identified 10 categories of needs from the data. However, how the need categories and the Orem model were related was unclear.

Harper (1984) applied the Orem model to nursing care of the elderly. Based on three self-care propositions inherent in the model, she hypothesized that 30 black, elderly, hypertensive women who received a medication self-care treatment program would show greater improvement on five health-related variables at 4 days and at 4 weeks posttreatment than would 30 black, elderly, hypertensive women who received a control teaching program. At 4 days, changes occurred in the hypothesized directions for knowledge, health locus of control, self-care medication behaviors, and medication error rates, but not for blood pressure; however, at 4 weeks this positive trend did not continue for any variable except knowledge of medication. This study was a good example of deducing hypotheses from the Orem propositions and then discussing the results in light of these propositions.

Using the Orem model, among other theoretical frameworks, Kubricht (1984) identified therapeutic self-care demands expressed by 30 adult outpatients undergoing external radiation therapy. The 30 subjects expressed 553 therapeutic self-care demands, with the largest percentage falling into the Orem universal self-care requisites of protection from hazards (20.4%), food and water (19.7%), and rest and activity (19.5%). Kubricht could have strengthened her study by clearly describing how she categorized data into the Orem universal self-care requisites and by establishing validity and reliability of her data collection tool.

In addition to research with patients, the Orem model was used to study families' reactions to children with cystic fibrosis (Kruger, Shawver, & Jones, 1980) and to compare knowledge, attitudes, confidence, and practice related to breast self-examination and self-care among nurses and nonnurses (Edgar, Shamian, & Patterson, 1984). In the former study, the Orem model was used to organize the theoretical perspective, sample, interview guide, and implications, whereas in the latter study the integration of the model throughout the study was less clear.

Finally, the Orem model was used specifically for tool construction. Kearney and Fleischer (1979) developed a tool consisting of 43 items that measured the Orem construct of exercise of self-care agency. Content and construct validity were established, as well as test-retest and split-half reliabilities. The investigators made a contribution to nursing science by operationalizing a key concept of the Orem model. Horn and Swain (1977) used the Orem model as the theoretical framework for a tool to measure outcomes of nursing care. The final tool, consisting of 348 valid and reliable outcome indices of quality nursing care, was comprehensive and represented a serious effort to organize an instrument for research purposes around a theoretical model of nursing. Despite this effort, only a few investigators (e.g., Hageman & Ventura, 1981; Harper, 1984) have used even a part of the tool in their research. Like Horn and Swain, Gallant and McLane (1979) also were interested in outcome criteria and developed a process for validation of a set of outcome criteria that was based partly on the Orem model.

RESEARCH BASED ON THE ROGERS SCIENCE OF UNITARY HUMAN BEINGS MODEL

In the Martha E. Rogers (Madrid & Winstead-Fry, 1986; Rogers, 1983) Science of Unitary Human Beings Models, persons and environments are viewed within four interrelated concepts: pattern, energy fields, four dimensionality, and open systems. The nature and direction of the relationship between the human and environmental fields are manifested through the principles of resonancy, helicy, and integrality (formerly complementarity). The nurse's role is to facilitate the patterning of unitary human beings and their environment to promote and maintain health.

In the early 1970s, Porter (1972a, 1972b) reported one of the earliest series of studies based on the Rogers model. Her hypothesis that infants who received planned passive cycling exercise would show significantly greater increases on six parameters of growth and development than infants who did not receive the exercises was supported. This study could have been strengthened by examining the study results in light of the Rogers model.

Fawcett (1977) also focused on the Rogers model but, in addition, extended the Rogers conceptualization of persons to families. Fawcett studied the relationship between time of pregnancy (during and after) and spouses' articulation of body concept and patterns of change in perceived body space. As with the Porter (1972a, 1972b) studies, this study could have been strengthened by examining the study results in light of the Rogers model and Fawcett's extension of the model. More recently, L. Smith (1983) referred to the Rogers model in exploring how families incorporated an adolescent mother and infant into the household; however, L. Smith did not describe how the model was used in the study.

Both Krieger (1974) and Quinn (1984) used the Rogers model, along with other pertinent literature, to study therapeutic touch. Krieger hypothesized that ill persons who received hand contact coupled with a strong intent to help or heal would show higher hemoglobin values than control persons who did not receive this treatment. Although the hypothesis was supported, the noncomparability of the experimental group (ill persons) and the control group (companions or family members of the ill persons) may have affected the results. Nevertheless, the Krieger study was a pioneering effort to bridge Eastern and Western health care, with some theoretical help from the Rogers model.

Building on the Krieger (1974) study and on the Rogers assumption that persons in interaction with other persons affect one another's energy fields, Quinn (1984) hypothesized that laying on of the hands was not necessary for healing to occur if other aspects of therapeutic touch such as centering, intent to heal, and noncontact moving of the hands over the body were followed. Her hypothesis was supported; hospitalized persons who received noncontact aspects of therapeutic touch, that is, all aspects of therapeutic touch were carried out except the laying on of the hands, reported less state anxiety than hospitalized persons who received a noncontact intervention that mimicked therapeutic touch, that is, the motions of therapeutic touch were mimicked, but noncontact therapeutic touch was not carried out. This study was a good example of theory testing although, as noted by Quinn, it did not validate directly the existence of an energy exchange.

A few investigators (Gill & Atwood, 1981; M. J. Smith, 1984; Tompkins, 1980) published research related to the Rogers concept of time or space-time. In her study of the effect of body dominance and restricted mobility on perceived duration of time, Tompkins briefly addressed the Rogers notion that the passage of time is part of the unidirectionality of life. In a study also involving restricted mobility (i.e., bed rest) and perceived duration of time, M. J. Smith used the Rogers model as part of her theoretical framework, although she did not address the model in her two earlier studies (1975, 1979) on bed rest and perceived duration of time. Using the Rogers principles of reciprocy (no longer in existence) and of helicy, with its space–time component, Gill and Atwood (1981) studied, among other concerns, the effect of epidermal growth factor (EGF) on the reepithelialization of epidermal excision wounds in a domestic pig. They found that as the concentration of EGF increased, so did the rate of the wounds' reepithelialization. However, Gill and Atwood were unable to finish their prearranged schedule of biopsies due to the pig's unexpected death from pulmonary congestion; thus, the long-term effect (through 48 hours) of the various concentrations of EGF could not be reported. Gill and Atwood not only described their perceptions of how the Rogers model related to the dependent variable, but they also used the principles of reciprocy and helicy to explain their study results. However, the extension of Rogers' beliefs about unitary human beings to animals has been questioned.

Goldberg and Fitzpatrick (1980) alluded to Rogers's principle of resonancy in their study of the effect of movement therapy, viewed as rhythmic pattern, on the morale and self-esteem of institutionalized elderly. Although not all their hypotheses were supported, they found that persons who participated in a movement therapy group showed significantly greater improvement in overall morale and in attitudes toward their own aging (a subscale of morale) than did persons who did not participate in the group. The authors appropriately concluded that these results lend some support to the Rogers model.

From a well-formulated premise based partly on the Rogers principles of resonancy and helicy, Floyd (1983) deduced the following theorem: Individuals experiencing a deviation in the rhythmic relationship with their environment will demonstrate more diversity and complexity in their sleep–wake patterns than will individuals not experiencing this deviation. From this theorem she further deduced several hypotheses that served as a basis for a study on rotating and nonrotating shift workers, and for a study on psychiatric inpatients and outpatients. Results of the shift worker study tended to support the theorem, whereas results of the clinical study did not. Floyd attributed this inconsistency to uncontrolled situational variables in the clinical study. A more plausible explanation is that inpatient hospitalization, although disruptive, does not usually cause a complete shift in the sleep–wake pattern as does shift rotation; therefore, the independent variable in the two studies was not comparable. In a derivative article, Floyd (1984) found that psychiatric inpatients slept significantly less than psychiatric outpatients, and that total sleep time of morning-type patients and evening-type patients was not significantly different.

RESEARCH BASED ON THE NEWMAN HEALTH MODEL

In Margaret A. Newman's model (1979), health is defined as expanded consciousness. The process of health is viewed through a series of interrelationships focusing on the concepts of time, space, movement, and consciousness. Time, space, and movement are seen as correlates of expanded consciousness and, thus, affect health. The nurse's role is to help people move toward higher levels of consciousness.

Unlike many other nurse theorists, Newman has published the majority of research related to her model of nursing. In sequential research (1972, 1976, 1982), she studied the concepts of movement and time. In her 1972 study, she investigated the effects of various walking rates on time estimation in 52 males and found no significant difference in estimated time perception based on walking rates. In this well-designed study, Newman carefully controlled for many extraneous variables. However, she placed no limit on how subjects estimated time (i.e., whether subjects used unconscious or conscious and compensatory timing mechanisms), nor did she discuss the rationale for and limitations in using only male subjects.

In the 1976 study, Newman replicated part of her 1972 study but, in addition, used predominantly female subjects and included types of compensatory timing mechanisms as an independent variable. Her primary hypothesis that preferred rate of walking would be related negatively to time estimation was not supported, neither under conditions of controlled compensation nor under conditions of freedom-to-compensate timing mechanisms. However, she found significant differences in time estimation in relation to two nonpreferred slower rates of walking.

In her 1982 study, Newman again studied the relationship between movement and time and, in addition, explored time as a developmental aspect of expanding consciousness with persons 60 to 88 years of age. None of the following hypotheses were supported: Perceived duration would be positively associated with age; older persons would manifest a higher index of consciousness (a comparison of the perceived passage of time to actual clock time) than younger persons; and preferred rate of walking would be associated positively with perceived duration. One of Newman's explanations for these findings was the insufficient variation of the time factor within the limited age range. However, her ancillary finding that time production estimates vary significantly by sex was important. It forced a reinterpretation of the data from her 1972 study where all subjects were male and her 1976 and 1982 studies where the subjects were predominantly female.

Recently Newman and Gaudiano (1984) hypothesized that depression would be negatively related to subjective time (perceived duration of the passage of time) in 68 elderly women. The women responded to a depression inventory and then were tested in regard to subjective time. The correlation between these two variables was 0.35, $p < .002$. The authors concluded that the hypothesis was supported, thus suggesting that depression masked increasing consciousness. However, the authors obtained no reliability data on the depression inventory, and the correlation between the variables, although significant, was not high.

M. J. Smith (1979, 1984), Tompkins (1980), and Engle (1984) also addressed the Newman research or model. M. J. Smith in her 1979 and 1984 replication studies focusing on processing of environmental stimuli and time estimation, described the results of the Newman 1976 study. In addition, in her 1984 study, Smith briefly noted the Newman thesis that health was an expansion of consciousness. Tompkins extended the Newman research in her study of the relationship between restricted or unrestricted joint movement and perceived duration of time. Consistent with the Newman findings, she found that restricted mobility significantly decreased perceived duration of time. Engle explicitly stated that she was testing propositions derived from the Newman model, although only the proposition that linked time as a function of movement was identified clearly. From this proposition, her hypothesis that cadence would be associated negatively with perceived duration of time in older female adults was supported. Other hypotheses related to self-assessment of health and personal tempo and to self-assessment of health and time perception were not supported. The Engle research not only built upon and supported the Newman research, but also expanded it by attempting to operationalize health. Although care was taken to ensure test–retest reliability for both personal tempo and time perception, Engle appropriately raised questions about (a) the validity of the tool used to operationalize health, and (b) the use of clock time to measure perception of time.

SUMMARY AND RESEARCH DIRECTIONS

Research related to five contemporary conceptual models of nursing has been summarized and assessed. Although the characteristics of the models vary (Jacobson, 1984), the strengths and weaknesses of the research as they relate to the models are similar.

Overall, strengths related to the research on the five reviewed models of nursing include demonstrations of: (a) the usefulness or potential usefulness of the models as an organizing framework for research, (b) the flexibility of the models in terms of breadth of clinical problems studied and of age groups addressed, and (c) the increasing sophistication of nurse investigators in testing hypotheses deduced from assumptions and propositions within the models.

Overall, gaps and weaknesses related to the research on the five reviewed models of nursing include: (a) the lack of integration of the models throughout the studies; (b) the little evidence either of systematic extension or replication of research based on nursing models; (c) the paucity of empirical validation of the models by the theorists who developed them; (d) the lack of explicit testing of assumptions and propositions within the models; (e) the lack of evidence to show how conceptual models of nursing used as frameworks for research influence nursing practice; and (f) the difficulty of retrieving studies based on nursing models when neither the theorist's name nor the name of the model appears in the study title or abstract.

Based on this summary, future research directions for nurse investigators include:

1. Clarify the relationships among conceptual models of nursing, nursing research, and nursing practice.
2. Design, replicate, and extend studies that focus on testing assumptions and propositions within the models.

3. Integrate the relevant components of the models throughout all appropriate phases of the research.
4. State explicitly the name of the theorist or the conceptual model in the title and abstract of research.
5. Consider use of a nursing model as a theoretical framework for research when the model is capable of structuring the study variables and explaining the study results.

By following these steps, the contribution of conceptual models of nursing to nursing research and practice will be enhanced. Through this enhancement, nursing science will be advanced.

REFERENCES

Allison, S. E. (1971). The meaning of rest: An exploratory nursing study. In *ANA clinical sessions* (pp. 191–205). New York: Appleton-Century-Crofts.

Bruce, G. L., Hinds, P., Hudak, J., Mucha, A., Taylor, M. C., & Thompson, C. R. (1980). Implementation of ANA's quality assurance program for clients with end-stage renal disease. *Advances in Nursing Science, 2*(2), 79–95.

Chang, B. L., Uman, G. C., Linn, L. S., Ware, J. E., Jr., & Kane, R. L. (1984). The effect of systematically varying components of nursing care on satisfaction in elderly ambulatory women. *Western Journal of Nursing Research, 6,* 367–379.

Damus, K. (1980). An application of the Johnson Behavioral System Model for nursing practice. In J. P. Riehl & C. Roy (Eds.), *Conceptual models for nursing practice* (2nd ed.) (pp. 274–289). New York: Appleton-Century-Crofts.

Derdiarian, A. K. (1983). An instrument for theory and research development using the Behavioral Systems Model for Nursing: The cancer patient. Part I. *Nursing Research, 32,* 196–201.

Derdiarian, A. K., & Forsythe, A. B. (1983). An instrument for theory and research development using the Behavioral Systems Model for Nursing: The cancer patient. Part II. *Nursing Research, 32,* 260–266.

Dickson, G. L., & Lee-Villasenor, H. (1982). Nursing theory and practice: A self-care approach. *Advances in Nursing Science, 5*(1), 29–40.

Dodd, M. J. (1982). Assessing patient self-care for side effects of cancer chemotherapy. Part I. *Cancer Nursing, 5,* 447–451.

Dodd, M. J. (1983). Self-care for side effects in cancer chemotherapy: An assessment of nursing interventions. Part II. *Cancer Nursing, 6,* 63–67.

Dodd, M. J. (1984). Measuring informational intervention for chemotherapy knowledge and self-care behavior. *Research in Nursing and Health, 7,* 43–50.

Edgar, L., Shamian, J., & Patterson, D. (1984). Factors affecting the nurse as a teacher and practicer of breast self-examination. *International Journal of Nursing Studies, 21,* 255–265.

Engle, V. F. (1984). Newman's conceptual framework and the measurement of older adults' health. *Advances in Nursing Science, 7*(1), 24–36.

Farkas, L. (1981). Adaptation problems with nursing home application for elderly persons: An application of the Roy Adaptation Nursing Model. *Journal of Advanced Nursing, 6*, 363–368.

Fawcett, J. (1977). The relationship between identification and patterns of change in spouses' body images during and after pregnancy. *International Journal of Nursing Studies, 14*, 199–213.

Fawcett, J. (1981a). Needs of cesarean birth parents. *JOGN Nursing, 10*, 372–376.

Fawcett, J. (1981b). Assessing and understanding the cesarean father. In C. F. Kehoe (Ed.), *The cesarean experience: Theoretical and clinical perspectives for nurses* (pp. 143–156). New York: Appleton-Century-Crofts.

Floyd, J. A. (1983). Research using Rogers' conceptual system: Development of a testable theorem. *Advances in Nursing Science, 5*(2), 37–48.

Floyd, J. A. (1984). Interaction between personal sleep–wake rhythms and psychiatric hospital rest–activity schedule. *Nursing Research, 33*, 255–259.

Gallant, B. W., & McLane, A. M. (1979). Outcome criteria: A process for validation at the unit level. *Journal of Nursing Administration, 9*(1), 14–21.

Gill, B. P., & Atwood, J. R. (1981). Reciprocy and helicy used to relate mEGF and wound healing. *Nursing Research, 30*, 68–72.

Goldberg, W. G., & Fitzpatrick, J. J. (1980). Movement therapy with the aged. *Nursing Research, 29*, 339–346.

Guzzetta, C. E. (1979). Relationship between stress and learning. *Advances in Nursing Science, 1*(4), 35–49.

Hageman, P. T., & Ventura, M. R. (1981). Utilizing patient outcome criteria to measure the effects of a medication teaching regimen. *Western Journal of Nursing Research, 3*, 25–33.

Hammond, H., Roberts, M. P., & Silva, M. C. (1983). The effect of Roy's first level and second level assessment on nurses' determination of accurate nursing diagnoses. *Virginia Nurse, 51*, 14–17.

Harper, D. C. (1984). Application of Orem's theoretical constructs to self-care medication behaviors in the elderly. *Advances in Nursing Science, 6*(3), 29–46.

Holaday, B. J. (1974). Achievement behavior in chronically ill children. *Nursing Research, 23*, 25–30.

Holaday, B. J. (1981). Maternal responses to their chronically ill infants' attachment behavior of crying. *Nursing Research, 30*, 343–348.

Holaday, B. J. (1982). Maternal conceptual set development: Identifying patterns of maternal response to chronically ill infant crying. *Maternal-Child Nursing Journal, 11*, 47–59.

Horn, B. J., & Swain, M. A. (1977). *Development of criterion measures of nursing care* (Vols. 1–2). Ann Arbor, MI: University of Michigan. (NTIS Nos. PB-267 004 and PB-267 005)

Ide, B. A. (1978). SPAL: A tool for measuring self-perceived adaptation level appropriate for a "well" elderly population. In E. E. Bauwens (Ed.)., *Clinical nursing research: Its strategies and findings* (pp. 56–63) (Monograph No. 2, Series 78). Indianapolis, IN: Sigma Theta Tau.

Jacobson, S. F. (1984). A semantic differential for external comparison of conceptual nursing models. *Advances in Nursing Science, 6*(2), 58–70.

Johnson, D. E. (1968). *One conceptual model for nursing.* Paper presented at Vanderbilt University School of Nursing, Nashville, TN.

Johnson, D. E. (1980). The Behavioral System Model for Nursing. In J. P. Riehl & C. Roy (Eds.), *Conceptual models for nursing practice* (2nd ed.) (pp. 207–216). New York: Appleton-Century-Crofts.

Karl, C. A. (1982). The effects of an exercise program on self-care activities for the institutionalized elderly. *Journal of Gerontological Nursing, 8,* 282–285.

Kearney, B. Y., & Fleischer, B. J. (1979). Development of an instrument to measure exercise of self-care agency. *Research in Nursing and Health, 2,* 25–34.

Kehoe, C. F. (1981). Identifying the nursing needs of the postpartum cesarean mother. In C. F. Kehoe (Ed.), *The cesarean experience: Theoretical and clinical perspectives for nurses* (pp. 85–141). New York: Appleton-Century-Crofts.

Krieger, D. (1974). The relationship of touch, with intent to help or heal [sic] to subjects' in vivo hemoglobin values: A study in personalized interaction. In American Nurses' Association (Ed.), *Ninth Nursing Research Conference* (pp. 39–58). Kansas City, MO: American Nurses' Association.

Kruger, S., Shawver, M., & Jones, L. (1980). Reactions of families to the child with cystic fibrosis. *Image, 12,* 67–72.

Kubricht, D. W. (1984). Therapeutic self-care demands expressed by outpatients receiving external radiation therapy. *Cancer Nursing, 7,* 43–52.

Leatt, P., Bay, K. S., & Stinson, S. M. (1981). An instrument for assessing and classifying patients by type of care. *Nursing Research, 30,* 145–150.

Leonard, C. V. (1975). Patient attitudes toward nursing interventions. *Nursing Research, 24,* 335–339.

Lewis, F. M., Firsich, S. C., & Parsell, S. (1979). Clinical tool development for adult chemotherapy patients: Process and content. *Cancer Nursing, 2,* 99–108.

Lovejoy, N. (1983). The leukemic child's perceptions of family behaviors. *Oncology Nursing Forum, 10*(4), 20–25.

Madrid, M., & Winstead-Fry, P. (1986). Rogers's conceptual model. In P. Winstead-Fry (Ed.), *Case studies in nursing theory* (pp. 73–102). New York: National League for Nursing.

Majesky, S. J., Brester, M. H., & Nishio, K. T. (1978). Development of a research tool: Patient indicators of nursing care. *Nursing Research, 27,* 365–371.

Miller, J. F. (1982). Categories of self-care needs of ambulatory patients with diabetes. *Journal of Advanced Nursing, 7,* 25–31.

Newman, M. A. (1972). Time estimation in relation to gait tempo. *Perceptual and Motor Skills, 34,* 359–366.

Newman, M. A. (1976). Movement tempo and the experience of time. *Nursing Research, 25,* 273–279.

Newman, M. A. (1979). *Theory development in nursing.* Philadelphia: F. A. Davis.

Newman, M. A. (1982). Time as an index of expanding consciousness with age. *Nursing Research, 31,* 290–293.

Newman, M. A., & Gaudiano, J. K. (1984). Depression as an explanation for decreased subjective time in the elderly. *Nursing Research, 33,* 137–139.

Nolan, M. R. G. (1977). Effects of nursing intervention in the operating room as recalled on the third postoperative day. In M. V. Batey (Ed.), *Communicating nursing research: Nursing research in the bicentennial year* (Vol. 9) (pp.

41–50). Boulder, CO: Western Interstate Commission for Higher Education.

Norris, S., Campbell, L. A., & Brenkert, S. (1982). Nursing procedures and alterations in transcutaneous oxygen tension in premature infants. *Nursing Research, 31*, 330–336.

Orem, D. E. (1971). *Nursing: Concepts of practice.* New York: McGraw-Hill.

Orem, D. E. (1980). *Nursing: Concepts of practice* (2nd ed.). New York: Mc-Graw-Hill.

Orem, D. E. (1985). *Nursing: Concepts of practice* (3rd ed.). New York: McGraw-Hill.

Porter, L. S. (1972a). Physical–physiological activity and infants' growth and development. In American Nurses' Association (Ed.), *Seventh nursing research conference* (pp. 1–43). New York: American Nurses' Association.

Porter, L. S. (1972b). The impact of physical–physiological activity on infants' growth and development. *Nursing Research, 21*, 210–219.

Quinn, J. F. (1984). Therapeutic touch as energy exchange: Testing the theory. *Advances in Nursing Science, 6*(2), 42–49.

Rogers, M. E. (1970). *An introduction to the theoretical basis of nursing.* Philadelphia: F. A. Davis.

Rogers, M. E. (1980). Nursing: A science of unitary man. In J. P. Riehl & C. Roy (Eds.), *Conceptual models for nursing practice* (2nd ed.) (p. 329–337). New York: Appleton-Century-Crofts.

Rogers, M. E. (1983). Science of unitary human beings: A paradigm for nursing. In I. W. Clements & F. B. Roberts (Eds.), *Family health: A theoretical approach to nursing care* (pp. 219–228). New York: Wiley.

Rothlis, J. (1984). The effect of a self-help group on feelings of hopelessness and helplessness. *Western Journal of Nursing Research, 6*, 157–169.

Roy, C. (1970). Adaptation: A conceptual framework for nursing. *Nursing Outlook, 18*, 42–45.

Roy, C. (1976). *Introduction to nursing: An adaptation model.* Englewood Cliffs, NJ: Prentice-Hall.

Roy, C. (1984). *Introduction to nursing: An adaptation model* (2nd ed.). Englewood Cliffs, NJ: Prentice-Hall.

Small, B. (1980). Nursing visually impaired children with Johnson's model as a conceptual framework. In J. P. Riehl & C. Roy (Eds.), *Conceptual models for nursing practice* (2nd ed.) (pp. 264–273). New York: Appleton-Century-Crofts.

Smith, C. E., Garvis, M. S., & Martinson, I. M. (1983). Content analysis of interviews using a nursing model: A look at parents adapting to the impact of childhood cancer. *Cancer Nursing, 6*, 269–275.

Smith, L. (1983). A conceptual model of families incorporating an adolescent mother and child into the household. *Advances in Nursing Science, 6*(1), 45–60.

Smith, M. J. (1975). Changes in judgment of duration with different patterns of auditory information for individuals confined to bed. *Nursing Research, 24*, 93–98.

Smith, M. J. (1979). Duration experience for bed-confined subjects: A replication and refinement. *Nursing Research, 28*, 139–144.

Smith, M. J. (1984). Temporal experience and bed rest: Replication and refinement. *Nursing Research, 33*, 298–302.

Tompkins, E. S. (1980). Effect of restricted mobility and dominance on perceived duration. *Nursing Research, 29*, 333–338.

Toth, J. C. (1980). Effect of structured preparation for transfer on patient anxiety on leaving coronary care unit. *Nursing Research, 29*, 28–34.

Index

Fitzpatrick, J. J., 47, 48
Fitzpatrick rhythm model, 48
Food intake regulation
  blood-borne substances in, 87
  caloric dilution and, 88

General pain indicies
  accuracy of, 27
  in nursing, 26–27
  verbal vs. nonverbal, 26–27
Glaser, E. M., 166
Goodrich, A. W., 179

Halberg, F., 55
Head nurses
  expectations for, 188–189
  leadership qualities of, perception of,
    188
  life goals of, longitudinal study of, 189
Health care professionals, clinical
    judgment ability in, 166
History, internal validity and, 14
Holland's Vocational Preference Inventory,
    use of, 182
Hospital Stress Rating Scale (HSRS), use
    of, 6–7
House, I. S., 142
Human biologic rhythms, 45–77
  circadian rhythms as, see Circadian
    rhythms
  literature review on, 45–46
  methodological matters in studying, 48–
    50
  nursing theory and, 47
Human performance
  body temperature and, 69
  circadian rhythms and, 68–70
  in nurses, 68–69
  sleep and, 68
Hypothalamus-pituitary-adrenocortical
    (HPA) system, response of, to stress
    and circadian rhythms, 93–95

Impact studies, on faculty practice in
    nursing, 147
Inadequate preoperational explication of
    constructs
  definition of, 11
  examples of, 11–12
  stress research and, 12
Indigenous health care practices, need for
    knowledge in, 218–219
Infant Activity Scale, use of, 52
Infant growth and development, Rogers
    model and, 237
Infarct size, prediction of, 81
Inferred degree of suffering
  in physical vs. psychological pain, 213–
    214
  study of, implications of, 214
  variables in, 213
Information processing theory, description
    of, 157–158

Informed consent, ethical issues and,124
Injection pain, interventions to relieve, 33–
    34
Institutionalized aged, care of
  alternative practices for, 212
  U.S. vs. Scottish approach to, 212
Intensive care unit (ICU)
  changes in, 107–108
  effectiveness of, 119–120
  environmental characteristics of, 110
  family impact of, 113–114; see also ICU
    stress in family
  nursing impact, 114–117; see also ICU
    stress in nursing
  patient impact, 108–113; see also ICU
    stress in patients
  mortality prediction in, 122–123
  prognosis prediction in, 121–122
  terminally ill care on, 121
Intensive care unit psychosis, study of,
    110–111
Intensive care unit stress in family
  and need perception, 113
  nursing interventions with, 114
  in various settings, 113–114
Intensive care unit stress in nursing, 114–
    117
  coping and, 116
  definitions of, 115
  interventions for, 116–117
  personality and, 115–116
  social supports in, 116
  sources of, 114–115
  and stress in other work environments,
    115
Intensive care unit stress in patients
  family involvement and, 111
  identification of, 109
  noise as, 109
  nursing interventions in, 112–113
  patient characteristics and, 110
  reduction of, 112
  research on, 110–112
  transfer preparation effects on, 112
Intensive care unit syndrome, study of,
    110–111
Internal validity
  definition of, 13
  history of, 14
  improvement of, 17
  selection and, 14
International nursing research
  assessment of, development of research
    tools for, 216–217
  comparability of samples in, 220–221
  cumulative investigation of, strategies
    for, 221–223
  data base for, 220
  definition of, 206–207
  ethics of, 221
  future research on, 219–221
  importance of, 210–211
  international organizations in, 220, 222

Contents from Volume I

Contents from Volume II

Contents from Volume III

Contents from Volume IV

ORDER FORM

Save 10% on Volume 6 with this coupon.

___Check here to order the ANNUAL REVIEW OF NURSING RESEARCH, Volume 6, 1988 at a 10% discount. You will receive an invoice requesting pre-payment.

Save 10% on all future volumes with a continuation order

___Check here to place your continuation order for the ANNUAL REVIEW OF NURSING RESEARCH. You will receive a pre-payment invoice with a 10% discount upon publication of each new volume, beginning with Volume 6, 1988. You may pay for prompt shipment or cancel with no obligation.

Name _____

Institution _____

Address _____

City/State/Zip _____

Examination copies for possible course adoption are available to instructors "on approval" only. Write on institutional letterhead, noting course, level, present text, and expected enrollment (Include $2.50 for postage and handling). Prices slightly higher overseas. Prices subject to change.

Mail this coupon to:
SPRINGER PUBLISHING COMPANY
536 Broadway, New York, N.Y. 10012